3 week

518.20233

KRO

D0347248

1015175

618 - 20233 KRO

Warrington Hospital Library

R04180

MIDWIFERY CARE
FOR THE FUTURE

4339501003098442772612

IN MEMORY OF LINDY

MIDWIFERY CARE FOR THE FUTURE

MEETING THE CHALLENGE

Edited by

Debra Kroll MSc, SRN, SCM, ADM, PGCEA

Senior Midwife, Obstetric Hospital, University College London
Hospitals NHS Trust, London

Baillière Tindall
London Philadelphia Toronto Sydney Tokyo

BAILLIÈRE TINDALL W.B. SAUNDERS
24–28 Oval Road
London NW1 7DX

The Curtis Center
Independence Square West
Philadelphia, PA 19106–3399, USA

Harcourt Brace & Company
55 Horner Avenue
Toronto, Ontario M8Z 4X6, Canada

Harcourt Brace & Company, Australia
30–52 Smidmore Street
Marrickville, NSW 2204, Australia

Harcourt Brace & Company, Japan
Ichibancho Central Building,
22–1 Ichibancho
Chiyoda-ku, Tokyo 102, Japan

© 1996 Baillière Tindall except for Chapter 6, pp. 98–123,
copyright © Judith Schott

This book is printed on acid-free paper

All rights reserved. No part of this publication may be reproduced,
stored in a retrieval system or transmitted, in any form or by any
means, electronic, mechanical, photocopying or otherwise, without
the prior permission of Baillière Tindall, 24–28 Oval Road, London NW1 7DX

A catalogue record for this book is available from the British Library

ISBN 0–7020–1758–2

Typeset by Phoenix Photosetting, Chatham, Kent
Printed in Great Britain by Hartnolls Ltd, Bodmin, Cornwall

Contents

List of Contributors

Carol Baxter Senior Lecturer, Faculty of Health, Department of Nursing Studies, University of Central Lancashire, Preston

Chris Ford General Practitioner, London

Jo Garcia Social Scientist, National Perinatal Epidemiology Unit, Radcliffe Infirmary, Oxford

Eileen Hutton President (1985–1995), The National Childbirth Trust, Bath

Steve Iliffe General Practitioner, London

Mavis Kirkham Professor of Midwifery, University of Sheffield, Sheffield

Debra Kroll Senior Midwife, Obstetric Hospital, UCLH NHS Trust, London

Sally Marchant Research Midwife, National Perinatal Epidemiology Unit, Radcliffe Infirmary, Oxford

Marianne Mead Principal Lecturer, Division of Midwifery and Child, University of Hertfordshire, Hatfield

Mary Newburn Head of Policy Research, The National Childbirth Trust, London

Judith Schott PROSPECT, London

Louise Silverton Director, Education and Practice Development, The Royal College of Midwives, London

Preface

Whenever I think of this book I think in terms of pregnancies and their gestation. It took more than three pregnancies for this book to reach full term. It started off as an embryo of an idea when it was obvious that community midwifery was altering dramatically and that those midwives based in the community were going to be at the forefront of change. However, as I started building up the ideas for a book dedicated to community midwifery practice, *Changing Childbirth* was published and it soon became clear that all midwives, wherever they practiced, were entering a whole new era of change. So every chapter was sought with all midwives in mind, those already qualified, those studying, those working in hospital, community and independent practice.

I am indebted to the many contributors to this book for their forebearance and perseverance and for giving me the opportunity to learn so much from them all, both in the pre-writing workshops and from the material in their chapters.

My special thanks go to Sarah James for her infinite patient and support when I wanted to give up. This was always available throughout and even during her two pregnancies. To her team, Robert Langham and Karen Gilmour, who helped keep the project afloat and were much better than me at persisting when chapters were late and reference material missing, my grateful appreciation.

I am indebted, as always, to Margot who continues to read my work with a critical eye and is always fair and encouraging, despite the fact that I still have not learnt to spell.

Finally, thanks to my friends, the pregnant women to whom I dedicate my career and to my family who never fail to remind me that it is all worthwhile. I am grateful to you all.

Introduction

It is often stated that one of the few things one can be sure about is change. It is an inherent part of our professional and everyday life. This book is essentially about change – change in health care provision, in society and in women's maternity care needs. It is about change brought about through research and education. But most of all it is about the challenge that all these changes pose for midwives and midwifery care.

The initial idea for this book emerged four and a half years ago before the Government Select Committee announced its findings and *Changing Childbirth* was published. It was already evident then that changes in the provision of maternity care were imminent.

The contributors come from a variety of backgrounds but they all share a commitment to women – centred care and the pivotal role of the midwife in this care.

The need to change the way pregnant women and their families are cared for during this important time in their lives is part of an enormous change in the culture of health care provision. This was reflected in the dissatisfaction voiced by women with the maternity services and the 'conveyor belt approach' to care. This dissatisfaction was a major stimulus for the setting up of the House of Commons Select Committee on Maternity Care and the resulting Expert Committee's report, *Changing Childbirth*.

Changing Childbirth gives midwives the opportunity to challenge current practices in midwifery care and organization. The aim of this book is not to provide a forum to discuss and debate *Changing Childbirth* – many texts have already been published addressing this. However, it is inevitable that the fundamental changes advocated by *Changing Childbirth* will have an impact on the subjects discussed in this book.

The NHS has been an integral part of health care provision since 1948. In the last few years health care in the NHS has been undergoing its most fundamental change since its inception. In Chapter 1 I discuss this 'new NHS' with its purchaser–provider split, hospital trusts and GP fundholders, and debate the effect it may have on the provision of maternity services in the future.

One of the main themes highlighted in *Changing Childbirth* is the importance of establishing women-centred maternity services and ensuring that these services meet the needs of those women for whom they are intended. The National Childbirth Trust has been championing the cause of pregnant women for many years. Eileen Hutton and Mary Newburn (Chapter 9) trace the origins and growth of the childbirth movement and the contribution that women have made to bringing about change in the organization of maternity care.

We live in a multicultural society and this is reflected nowhere better than in the maternity services. Carol Baxter (Chapter 2) describes this multiethnic, multicultural society and some of the problems and inequalities in health care experienced by women from the ethnic minorities. She argues for the recognition of the needs of all women and for an ethnically sensitive maternity service. She offers a useful tool to assist readers to evaluate their own attitudes, knowledge and skills around the issues of racism and ethnic sensitivity.

Change is a slow and, for some, a very difficult process. This is why it is vital to assist change and understand the stress it may cause to many working in the field of health care provision. Judith Schott (Chapter 6) considers the carers, the midwives. As she so clearly points out, the needs of health care professionals are seldom prioritized. Although there is a wealth of material documenting the effect of stress on nurses, very few authors have addressed the needs of midwives as they undergo major changes in the way they practice and provide care.

The education and preparation of midwives is of paramount importance to meet the challenges of future maternity care. Midwifery education has itself undergone major transformation in the last few years. Schools of midwifery are no longer an integral part of a maternity unit. Many have moved into institutes of higher education allowing midwives to graduate with a registerable qualification jointly validated by the National Boards for Nursing, Midwifery and Health Visiting and an institute of higher education. Louise Silverton (Chapter 5) debates this move, and its advantages and disadvantages, as well as the impact it has had on service provision.

Midwife means 'with woman'. Throughout history midwives have been part of the social group they served. This is no longer the case in this country. The move from home to hospital birth, the fragmentation of care and the professionalization of midwifery have served to separate midwives from women. Mavis Kirkham (Chapter 8) describes this move away from the community base and examines what is happening as midwives strive to go back to 'being with women'.

Interprofessional care and collaboration is the buzz word of the 90s. Many professionals have an input into maternity care. Some of this input is considered necessary and some regarded as a duplication and therefore a waste of resources. Chris Ford and Steve Iliffe (Chapter 3), two inner city general practitioners, look at interprofessional collaboration in community-based maternity care. They discuss the importance of good communication and liaison between the three professionals involved in maternity care: midwives, general practitioners and obstetricians. They question the education received by senior house officers (SHO) and whether this is truly the way to prepare them for maternity care in the primary health care setting. A simple checklist is suggested for purchasing community-based maternity care.

Postnatal care is often viewed as the Cinderella of maternity care. Much emphasis is placed on antenatal and intrapartum care ignoring the potential of postnatal care. The way postnatal care is provided has changed much in recent years. While some practitioners advocate extending the midwife's role in the postnatal period, others question whether we really know what the purpose of postnatal care is. Jo Garcia and Sally Marchant (Chapter 4) look at the background to postnatal care and describe the variety of visiting policies across the country. Their chapter concludes with some suggestions for audit and evaluation of this important aspect of care.

Research has been fundamental in moving midwifery practice forward. It forms a significant part of midwifery education and underlies practice and development. In order to bring about change based on research it is important to be critical and analytical when reading research findings. Marianne Mead (Chapter 7) provides readers with an introduction to the concepts of research and a taste for research which she hopes may inspire readers to go on and become midwifery researchers themselves.

This book highlights many issues that will provide a challenge to midwives planning and providing care now and in the future. It is, however, by no means exhaustive. Many issues have not been addressed. Amongst these are changing family structures, HIV and its influence on maternity care provision, the legal aspects pertaining to maternity care, risk management and the future of supervision in midwifery, to name but a few.

Change is often viewed as the move from a steady state to one of uncertainty. In maternity care it must be seen as an opportunity and a challenge to make a difference in the way midwives provide care. It is what many women have been asking for and what many midwives have been trying to provide for a long time, often unsupported. Debates and discussions about how and where maternity care is provided, and by whom, will continue for many years to come. I hope this book goes some way to contributing to the debate.

Debra Kroll

1

Working for Women: Assessing Needs, Planning Care

Debra Kroll

INTRODUCTION

Every pregnant women has unique needs relating not only to her medical and obstetrical history but also derived from her ethnic, cultural, social and family background. The aim of a modern maternity service as set out in *Changing Childbirth* (Department of Health (DoH) 1993b) is to recognize the characteristics of the local population and ensure that the services are appropriate, sensitive and accessible to all women who use them.

This chapter will explore how the needs of pregnant women and their families can be translated to provide a safe and effective maternity service. It will examine the ways in which providers can work together with purchasers to assess needs and provide the best quality maternity care.

It is not the remit of this chapter to go into extensive detail about the organization of the National Health Service (NHS). This is available in other texts. However a brief understanding of the most recent health service reforms will help to put the chapter into context.

The National Health Service today

The last decade of health care has been one of major change, not just in the understanding of the epidemiology of diseases but in the structure and functioning of the health care services. One of the greatest strengths of the NHS, and one which has endured since its inception in 1948, is the concept of responsibility for the health of geographically defined populations, not just patients who seek help from the service (Donaldson and Donaldson 1993). A framework of service provision helps to ensure that a comprehensive range of services based in general practice, hospital and in the community is available to local populations on the basis of their health needs.

The latest major organizational change in the NHS took place following the National Health Service and Community Care Act (1990). The implementation of a system of purchasers and providers of health care formed the cornerstone of the White Paper *Working for Patients* (Secretaries of State for Social Services, Wales, Northern Ireland and Scotland 1989a). Under the new system the purchasing or commissioning agencies are charged with the task of determining the health care needs of the local population and purchasing health care to meet these needs. These agencies are separated statutorily from those responsible for providing health services.

This differs from the old system in which the same institution (primarily within the NHS) assessed the care needs of individuals and provided treatment rationed in accordance with the institution's local priorities (Wilson and McAnulty 1991). Under the new system purchasers are encouraged to shop around for the best deal for their clients. The role of the providers, essentially all hospitals, hospital trusts and community units, is to ensure that their services meet the requirements set out in the purchaser's contracts.

The introduction of the competitive market was intended to relieve and eventually eradicate the economic and structural problems that inhibit the delivery of an efficient and personalized health service (Bradshaw and Bradshaw 1994).

Previously the health service has always been driven by the providers. The reformed service aims to reduce central control and permit local consumers to govern competition. In theory the system aims to permit patient choice. However, many would argue that patients seldom had a choice in the past and the new system is too complex to allow choice in the true sense of the word. Hospital services, including maternity care, are purchased by the District Health Authority (DHA), often in conjunction with the local Family Health Service Authority (FHSA). This joint commissioning agency effectively represents the consumer. This, according to some authors, allows minimal consumer empowerment and leaves the reformed system as paternalistic as ever (Bradshaw and Bradshaw 1994).

Another of the NHS reforms allows GP practices with more than 9000 patients to apply for fundholding status. Some practices are large enough to do this on their own while other smaller practices have joined together for the purpose of applying to become joint fundholders. Practices that hold their own budget can decide how best to spend their allocated funds within certain areas. They can 'shop around' and purchase certain outpatient and diagnostic services and some inpatient and day treatment. At present GP fundholders cannot purchase maternity care. This is done by the Health Authority on behalf of the total local population. However, it is not clear whether this will remain the case in the future. There is a strong belief that GP fundholders, as part of their bid to assert more power in the internal market, will begin to provide a much wider range of services including maternity care (Tyler and Jenkins 1994).

This fundamental change in the way GPs practise means that fundholding practices will in effect be both purchasers and providers of health care services. This raises serious questions as to whether the services provided will be in the best interest of the people for whom it is intended.

At the time of writing this chapter, change was in the air once more. Primary legislation allowing the abolition of DHAs and FHSAs and the creation of new Health Authorities was coming before Parliament. Subject to receiving Royal Assent, The Health Authorities Bill will allow the new Health Authorities to be established on 1 April 1996. This will create a single authority at local level with responsibility for implementing national health policy. It is expected to promote the involvement of GPs in purchasing by developing increasingly primary care led purchasing.

Some of the functions previously invested with Regional Health Authorities will be transferred to the new Health Authorities. One of the most important to midwifery practice is supervision of midwives. The Health Authorities will act as the local supervising authority for midwives under the Nurses, Midwives and Health Visitors Act (1979).

ASSESSING HEALTH NEEDS: WHERE TO BEGIN?

The task of the purchasing or commissioning agencies is to determine the health care needs of local populations and purchase health care to meet these needs. The assessment of a population's needs is not a straightforward process. Health is not easily defined, other than in broad terms, i.e. the absence of disease, and it cannot be measured with exactness. The interpretations of need centre around such concepts as demand, want, requirement and necessity. The Shorter Oxford Dictionary expands on this by defining need as a matter requiring action to be taken. The key to assessing the health care needs of a population is the ability first to assess the health status of the given population and then translate this into a statement of needs (Connah and Pearson 1991). Health needs can be defined as that which a person requires to stay in good health and the known ability to benefit from the health care provided. The former includes employment, nutrition, housing and access to social and health care services.

Many different processes to assess needs are required to underpin the contracting process (Editorial 1992). A wide range of data are available to demonstrate the health of the population living in a particular place, its size and composition, the people's lifestyle, the illness and diseases experienced in that population and the number of births and deaths. By piecing together data of different types it is possible to begin to develop an understanding of the health of a population.

The separation of those responsible for providing health care from those responsible for purchasing services is based on the assumption that commissioning agencies would be able to contract services on the basis of their assessment of local population health care needs. It gives purchasers the opportunity to focus on improving the health services for the local population through the contracting process. However, there are still major obstacles in defining and measuring health care needs.

Theoretically it ought to be possible to arrive at a statement of the absolute need of a population (Connah and Pearson 1991). However, this is almost impossible as it would require a statement of health of every member of the population, which would be costly, impractical and out of date before it was completed. Therefore a population's needs represent the aggregate of the needs of many individuals.

Despite the fact that health needs assessment is a complex task, the concept is not difficult to understand. Bailey (personal communication) constructs the following scenario to demystify the process and I will draw on this to explain the process further. Since this book is about the provision of care for pregnant women I will use Bailey's scenario to explore the maternity services.

Imagine that you are a midwife who has been put on a desert island and told to ensure that a maternity service exits. What would you need to do?

The first task is to find out about the women on the island for whom you are going to provide a service. You would need to know the number of women of childbearing age on the island and whether this population was predicted to grow or decrease. You would need to know about the health of the women on the island, and whether there were any endemic diseases on the island. You would need to find out how many women and babies died during childbearing, whether this was better or worse in some parts of the island and whether there were any factors that could be attributed to the mortality and morbidity rates. You would be interested to know whether the government or tribes had influence over this factor/or had tried to do anything about it. You would also need to find out whether there were any particular cultural or religious traditions and taboos around childbearing.

Your next task would be to find out what type of services existed on the island for pregnant women. Who provided the service and where was it located? Was it local or centralized and did women have to travel to it or did it travel to them? Importantly, the wishes of the women would be paramount. What kind of maternity service did they want? Were they happy with what existed and did it meet their needs? You would need to investigate the history of the service, and whether it was influenced by the island's government (if there was one) or particular tribes. Finally, you would need to find out how much it costs to run.

Donaldson and Donaldson (1993) draw a distinction between 'health related' and 'health service' data. Health related data refer primarily to demographic data, while health service data refer to the use that a population makes of health services. Both are significant for the provision of maternity services. Health related data provide information about the age of the population, i.e. the number of women of childbearing age, the number of births and deaths, the age of mothers at the time of birth, etc. Health service data give information about the use of the maternity services, e.g. which hospitals and which community-based clinics are used.

However, all health data are subject to quantitative and qualitative deficiencies which limit the conclusions that can be drawn from them. They do none the less provide a basis from which to plan care.

The first part of the above scenario represents an epidemiological approach to health needs assessment. This requires information about the local population, patterns of disease, the costs and effectiveness of provision and the quality of care. An ideal approach would be to conduct epidemiological surveys to establish the incidence and prevalence of key diseases to establish the proportion of the population that has been treated and needs treatment. In Britain the principal way to obtain this information is through the Offices of Population Census and Surveys (OPCS), which provides data about the population, its size and composition. In order to provide this data a periodic count of the characteristics of a population in a given area is conducted. Known as a population census, it is enshrined in law and carried out every 10 years by the OPCS.

Population estimates, produced yearly, provide statements of population size and details of characteristics such as age and sex for periods between census points. This is derived by taking the census as a baseline and adding births, subtracting deaths and making allowances for migration. A legal requirement to register births and deaths makes it simple to obtain this information and provides fairly sound estimates. Migration, particularly internal (within a country), is more difficult to predict. Midwives working in inner city areas will be familiar with the problems of a mobile population, particularly in areas where there is a high density of bed and breakfast accommodation, a roofless population and travellers. Population projections are attempts to forecast the size and characteristics of the population into the future making assumptions about fertility, mortality and migration.

Health service activity data

To find out about service provision in Britain, health service activity data must be examined. Almost all activity in the health service is covered by some form of aggregated data collection. These data are used to judge service usage and performance. Readers will be familiar with Kroner returns, one of the main systems for recording health service activity.

Information on birthweights has implications for neonatal and postnatal services and will also influence perinatal mortality rates and therefore is also important when assessing service needs. A variety of indices of fertility can be obtained including general fertility rates and age-specific fertility rates. The latter is useful in assessing whether, in a given population, there are more babies born to teenage mothers or older women.

An important means of assessing health needs is to examine government reports which give information on morbidity and mortality in mothers and children. This can be obtained primarily from two sources. The triennial *Report on Confidential Enquiries into Maternal Deaths in The United Kingdom* analyses details of almost every maternal death. Practice is assessed in respect of each case. The report identifies causes of death and the trends in incidence. It discusses substandard care and makes recommendations.

Confidential Enquiries into Stillbirths and Deaths in Infancy (CESDI) is a relatively new activity. Since 1991 all Regional Health Authorities (RHAs) have been required to establish a review of stillbirths and neonatal deaths within their population. In addition, since 1993, RHAs have been required to participate in the national CESDI. The national survey gives important information on perinatal mortality and will, in the future, allow for national overview and comparisons. Information on infant morbidity can be obtained from the OPCS, which runs a national monitoring system on the frequency of congenital malformations and other fetal abnormalities in the population.

There are many other ways in which purchasers can be guided about the services they wish to purchase. Many national and professional guidelines and reports are available. Some examples are the various documents from the United Kingdom Central Council for Nursing Midwifery and Health Visiting (UKCC) and the Department of Health. Other reports can be of value. Important Select Committee reports will influence the process of purchasing relevant care. The most recent and important one for the midwifery services was *Changing Childbirth* (DoH 1993b). It is important to remember that these indicators are not targets that must be met, but rather a means of guiding purchasers and providers in planning future services.

Research and audit play a significant part in informing health policy and clinical decisions. Purchasers will be aware of the Cochrane Pregnancy and Childbirth database, a part of the Cochrane Database of Systematic Reviews, which provides information on the effects of health care. The Cochrane Pregnancy and Childbirth Database is the first specialized Cochrane database. The evidence that resulted from the first collection of reviews on specific topics was published in a two volume book *Effective Care in Pregnancy and Childbirth* (Chalmers *et al.* 1989). The database is updated regularly and is now available on disk. Some of the research topics in these two volumes lend themselves to audit; examples are the use of different perineal suture material, steroids in preterm labour and external cephalic version for breech presentation.

Visits to, and reviews of, local services and a review of complaints are other means of providing commissioning agencies with information to support the purchasing process. Both purchasers and providers will be influenced by media coverage, particularly with regard to local issues.

Obtaining the views of the consumer

Often there is a difference in perception of need between consumers and medical professionals. The realistic way of assessing need means that statistical estimates are translated, using science and art, into an assessment of health care needs. Practically, provision of services must be related to what women will accept and what the health service can provide.

Assessing needs from the consumer point of view can be achieved through consultation, surveys, consumer 'storytelling' and consumer focus groups on specific topics. Local surveys are one consumer approach by which local needs can be determined. Involving the consumers acknowledges the importance of gauging the community's perception of its own priorities. If care is to be women–centred, the views of the users of maternity services in the planning and delivery of care are vital.

In theory it should be easy to determine the needs of a population by local surveys (Bowling 1992, Gillam 1992). Most research projects examining maternity services include some aspect of consumer satisfaction. There is a growing belief that the qualitative data obtained from research projects are as important as the quantitative results in influencing health care policy (Martin 1990). Manuals specifically designed to assist Health Authorities and other researchers to gain the views of women using maternity services have been designed (Mason 1989).

The needs assessment process therefore involves a variety of approaches including the use of routinely available data to provide continuous surveillance of health patterns and trends, *ad hoc* analysis of routinely available data to answer a particular problem or address a particular question and the gathering of data that are not routinely available (Donaldson and Donaldson 1993). Alongside this, data establishing the views of consumers are imperative in the decision-making process about health care needs. Each purchasing authority must make its own projections.

Bowling (1992) raises some pertinent questions about the process of assessing health care needs that will continue to be debated for some time as the purchasing of services is developed:

- What are health needs?
- Whose definition or value judgement can be used?
- How can estimates of need be translated into practice?
- How can quantity of care needed be balanced against quality of care provided?
- How can conflicting health priorities be resolved?
- What research methods and instruments should be used?

PRACTICAL APPROACHES TO MATERNITY SERVICES NEEDS ASSESSMENT

The World Health Organization (WHO) defines health as 'physical, mental and social well-being, not merely the absence of disease or infirmity'. This definition has particular significance when assessing the needs of the pregnant (or those planning or potentially able to be pregnant) local population. Pregnancy is not an illness. For most women it is a normal physiological process. A small minority have complications and these have to be accounted for when assessing the need for different types of maternity care.

If, as many believe, the strength of our society is based on good parenting within stable families, the investment in high-quality maternity services is a cornerstone of sound economics (Connah and Pearson 1991). It is of vital importance to remember that the task of assessing health care needs is not only the responsibility of the purchasers but also of the providers, who need to ensure that they are meeting the requirements of those purchasing and using their services.

The questions raised in the desert island scenario that I used earlier to describe how purchasers can go about assessing the needs of pregnant women can be similarly used by the providers of maternity services when reviewing their service provision. It would include three broad stages: firstly, an assessment of what currently exists, i.e. what services are currently provided; secondly, finding out what women who use the services want, and finally, something which may not be an issue on a desert island, mapping out the total maternity services provided by the unit and those of neighbouring health authorities and maternity units. This mapping exercise will include information about the availability of home deliveries in all areas and the location of local GPs who are prepared to support home deliveries. It would also examine what community midwifery services are available, e.g. community-based antenatal care, team midwifery, midwife beds, DOMINO deliveries, etc. The availability of waterbirths and alternative therapies may be important if that is what local women want.

We have seen that any assessment of need requires a definition of the population for which the service is required. It is also the responsibility of the provider units to ensure that they have detailed population profiles which will allow accurate assessment of the childbearing population that will require their services. Important aspects that need assessing are the local ethnic mix, the numbers of homeless and unsupported families and the numbers of teenage as well as older childbearing women. Each of these has particular needs.

It is important for midwives working in the local community to build up a community profile. This is one practical way of providing a picture of the community in which the women and their families live and the midwives will work. It is not only important to gain information about the population groups but also the resources and services already available within the community. These include statutory and voluntary resources, cultural and community support services and pressure groups set up particularly to address maternity issues. Liaising with these groups will bring midwives into direct contact with the leaders of the community and lead to a better understanding of the local community. It is important to approach these groups when seeking lay or local representation on working parties to address particular issues in the provision of care. It is often simpler to opt for representation from consumer groups that are more vocal, e.g. the National Childbirth Trust. However, this group may not be a true representative of the local community.

Marketing the service

Once services are set up it is important to ensure that users and potential users get to know about them. Advising local GPs about the variety of maternity services available and keeping them up to date with changes is an important part of marketing. A community profile will highlight areas where it is important to advertise the services, e.g. the local health centre, family planning centre, temporary accommodation and cultural centres where women may meet. It is important to ensure that services are advertised in appropriate languages, are acceptable in each place and will not cause offence to any one group.

Informing local women of the services available is important both if the maternity unit is the only one in the locality and if it is competing with other maternity units in the area. Some purchasing authorities, working together with local provider units, compile information booklets outlining all the local services available for each specialty. Maternity care booklets could specify the variety of services, particularly community-based services, offered by each local maternity unit, the location of GPs happy to support home births, what tests were offered by each provider unit, etc.

Maternity units that provide services to women who come from several health authorities must carefully assess their services to ensure they meet the needs of both these women and local women. There may be a tendency to plan services to meet the particular needs of the host purchaser, without considering whether these are acceptable to women from other areas.

CONSUMER CHOICE

Needs assessment must be linked to outcome. The effect on health of care provided is an important test of whether the needs assessment was right and whether health can be improved through the services contracted. In maternity care neonatal and maternal morbidity and mortality is an important measure of success. However, with enormous improvements in the safety of childbirth and a great reduction in maternal and neonatal deaths, demands for a better service concentrate on improvements in service. Maternity services must be more user friendly and acknowledge the individual needs of pregnant women and their families. Continuity of care, choice, control and accessible care now dominate the list of demands of childbearing women. These soft outcomes are not always easy to measure.

A woman's choice, in particular with regard to which hospital she wishes to attend for her antenatal care and delivery, is not always evident in the new reformed NHS. The GP is still the first port of call for most women when they discover they are pregnant. The GP will refer the women to the hospital where the local purchasing authority has a contract. At present this includes fundholding practices, which cannot purchase maternity care. If a woman chooses a maternity unit that has no contract with her purchasing authority, her referral has to be dealt with as an extra-contractual referral (ECR). It is then the decision of the purchasing authority whether the woman's choice can be accommodated. If there is no particular medical or obstetric reason for a woman to be at the hospital of her choice, the purchasing authority may effectively deny her the choice by refusing to pay for the care. Without an agreed ECR no woman can receive any care and this can prove distressing to pregnant women and cause concern to maternity services as vital screening tests may be delayed or missed whilst the purchasers and providers negotiate over the ECR.

Purchasing authorities set a certain amount of funding aside for necessary ECRs. Since most purchasing authorities have contracts with more than one maternity unit, they may argue that (within reason) choice is on offer. ECRs are expensive and purchasing authorities may feel that funds set aside should be used for urgent cases where sick patients may have to be cared for in specialized units.

SERVICE SPECIFICATIONS

Service specifications are a vehicle for explaining the health needs, wishes and requirements of a local population and translating them into a contractual arrangement.

They are used by purchasers, as part of the contracting process, to specify particular services that they would like to see provided by the provider units. These may include the availability of services in the community, specific screening tests, information in various languages and a variety of quality issues, e.g. waiting times and privacy. The service specification may vary according to the specialty. In many cases there is a specification to cover the specialty as well as general specifications that cover all specialties within the provider unit. These usually encompass quality and standards.

Health Authorities base their standards on the Patient's Charter (DoH 1992), local patients' charters and on Maxwell's six dimensions of health care quality: accessibility, appropriateness to need, efficiency, effectiveness and accessibility of services (Maxwell 1984). There is usually a section on the handling of complaints.

Service specifications for maternity services must be based on up-to-date knowledge of research and changing practice. In recent years various documents have been published advising Health Authorities and commissioning agencies on the purchasing of maternity care (North East Thames RHA 1992, Welsh Health Planning Forum, 1991).

Following the publication of the Select Committee's report on Maternity Services (1992) the Government set up the Expert Maternity Group to 'review policy on NHS maternity care, particularly during childbirth, and make recommendations' (Maternity Services: Government Response 1992). Its recommendations, published in *Changing Childbirth* (DoH 1993b), are now acknowledged as Government policy on maternity care. *Changing Childbirth* clearly lays out the type of services it wished to see for pregnant women within 5 years of publication. It concentrates on the key components to achieve a women–centred service which meets the needs of the women for whom the service is intended.

The Expert Maternity Group recognized the need for both purchasers and providers to be involved in the process. Each key objective is highlighted by action points for purchasers and providers. This gives all those purchasing maternity care for the local population an ideal basis from which to start when looking at the available services and what to specify for the future.

The Patient's Charter: Maternity Services (DoH 1994) is part of the departments review of the maternity services. It sets out the rights and standards of services that apply to maternity care. It embraces some of the key points of *Changing Childbirth* (DoH 1993b) focusing on the named midwife, specific times for appointments and limits on waiting times, choice of labour companion and the right of every woman to see and carry her own maternity notes.

THE CONTRACTING PROCESS

Clause 4 of the NHS and Community Care Act (1990) covers NHS contracts. The contract is the means through which the purchasers of care secure a particular level and quality of services from hospitals and other providers of care for its population.

The contracting process should be seen as an opportunity to discuss and agree how improvements in patient care can be achieved and over what time period. The start of each contracting year begins when contracts are signed and preparations begin for planning the next year's activities. The onset of this rolling process is the evaluation by purchasers and providers of the effects of the previous year's contract (Coates 1994). The contracts are drawn up following discussion and negotiation between the purchasing authority and the provider unit. Evaluation and monitoring of health service provision must be on a continuous basis and agreed on in the service contract.

There are three broad types of contracts for purchasing clinical services. The first and most general is the *block contract*. In this contract the purchasing authority agrees with a hospital or other health care provider that a payment will be made to enable patients to have access to a defined range of services. Specifications may be made about the quality of services. Funding is provided by regular instalments from the commissioning agencies irrespective of the actual use of the facilities. Most maternity contracts still fall into this group. This type of contract has the advantage of simplicity. It allows the provider the flexibility to handle unexpected fluctuations in the number of cases treated. The disadvantage is that it is difficult for the purchaser to monitor quality and to ensure that maximum value for money is being obtained. It relies on the provider to ensure contract specifications are met. For the provider the main disadvantage is that the number of cases presenting for treatment within the contract may exceed expectation and available resources. This contract tends to be used when information systems are weak and monitoring the volume of work is difficult, or in situations where predicting the volume of work is problematic.

The second type of contract is more specific and is called the *cost and volume contract*. In this type of contract the purchaser agrees with the provider that a particular volume of work will be dealt with and the two parties fix a price. The contract includes quality criteria. The advantage of this contract is that there is a greater degree of certainty on the part of the purchaser in the amount of work that will be carried out. The provider also knows the volume of work with which it will need to cope. This type of contract is popular as it is open to negotiation. It may have a clause that allows for extra work to be carried out at a marginal cost.

The third and most specific type of contract is the *cost per case contract*. The cost of each case is specified to the purchaser, reflecting the severity of the health problem. The particular advantage to the purchaser is that it enables the best price to be obtained for the specified category of care. It tends to be used for isolated cases where the patients are treated outside of their district of residence and their home district health authority is subsequently invoiced.

A contract is divided into several areas. A typical contract contains an introduction which includes a summary of the service, what is being contracted for and with which provider. The aims and objectives of the service provision are specified in the next section and this is usually followed by a précis of the local population. The volume to be contracted for is specified. The terms of the contract are usually for 1 year and payment terms are specified. Every contract has a section on quality guidelines. The purchaser agrees indicators that it will monitor and use in future discussions when new contracts are set. Finally, specific quality issues are highlighted. In maternity care, examples include the purchaser's request that all women are offered the double test to screen for their risk of spina bifida and Down's syndrome.

Purchasing health care on behalf of a local population is a still a relatively new activity. In the past those purchasing maternity services tended to use historic demand as a basis for contracting, and for the immediate future, until more sophisticated tools are developed, it is likely that needs will be assessed and services purchased on the basis of the previous year's data. This was demonstrated by the conclusions drawn by a small study team set up with the remit:

. . . to consider examples of good practice in commissioning and providing maternity services in units led by midwives and/or general practitioners; and to report its conclusions.

(DoH, 1993a).

The team made a series of visits to several maternity units. They aimed for a range of examples of organizations and care. They concluded that almost all the service developments examined were initiated by providers. Purchasers were still at an early stage in thinking about commissioning maternity services. However, all recognized the potential of contracting as a process for influencing the range and quality of services.

Bradshaw and Bradshaw (1994) believe that the absence of sufficiently sophisticated purchasing tools has led to a managed market characterized by price fixing. This is very evident in the purchase of maternity care. Maternity contracts still tend to be block contracts with little differentiation for the variety of care on offer and the type of delivery. In reality the cost of high-risk pregnancy care, which requires consultant obstetric, medical and anaesthetic input and a Caesarean operation, is the same as the care of a woman who has had a problem-free pregnancy, community-based midwifery care, a normal delivery and 1 day in hospital postnatally.

Meaningful assessment of needs is the key to successful purchasing and provision of care. Yet to date the health needs of a population have rarely been assessed in ways that are useful to health service managers and planners (Gillam 1992). There are few solid or reliable data on the cost of various types of maternity services. Limited information exists in the area of health economics.

Successful purchasing requires the ability to focus on consumer needs, and to challenge the appropriateness of current services offered by providers. Midwives are well placed to do this, yet few health purchasing teams include a practising midwife. The contracting process appears to be handled by financiers and contracting departments, and midwives on the 'shop floor' of the provider units are often unaware of the process involved and the service that they are, in effect, 'being signed up' to provide.

Now that purchasing systems are in place, purchasers of maternity care are in a position to be more proactive and to seek to influence the range and quality of services available to pregnant women and their families. However, it appears that there is still some way to go before this becomes truly visible.

WORKING TOGETHER

Purchasing health care is a multidisciplinary activity and includes providers and users. The needs assessment process involves a variety of approaches including the use of routinely available data to provide continuous surveillance of health patterns and trends, *ad hoc* analysis of routinely available data to answer a particular problem or address a particular question and the gathering of data that is not routinely available (Donaldson and Donaldson 1993). Alongside this, data establishing the views of consumers are imperative in the decision-making process about health care needs.

In a consumer-led service the voice of its users needs to be heard. The formal acceptance of *Changing Childbirth* (DoH 1993b) marks the beginning of a new era when all maternity services will become more responsive to women's needs (Lewinson 1994).

Delivering an appropriate service to women who may not be able, or do not have the opportunity, to articulate their needs is a big challenge to the maternity services. One of the arguments put forward against a women-centred service in principle is that women may find it difficult to express their needs. They may lack practice in identifying needs, lack confidence in articulating them, or have a low self-esteem and no expectations that those providing maternity care will be particularly interested in them (Perkins 1991). The new order for cooperative working requires consumers to work closely with both purchasers and providers in every arena to ensure that maternity services are readily accessible and acceptable to women and sensitive to the needs of the local community.

Decisions about the ways in which maternity care is organized have an important influence on the sort of care that women receive. Despite the fact that the internal market was introduced in the interest of avoiding conflict, it is impossible to provide a safe and effective maternity service without close cooperation and communication between those responsible for providing the care that is to be purchased by those responsible for assessing needs.

Maternity services liaison committee

> . . . *to give people an effective voice in the shaping of the health services locally will call for a radically different approach from that employed in the past. In particular, there needs to be a move (away from one-off consultation)* . . . *towards on going involvement of local people in the purchasing activities*
> (National Health Services Management Executive 1992)

We have seen that needs assessment is the joint responsibility of purchasers and providers of care. The Maternity Services Liaison Committees (MSLC) provides an ideal forum for this task. This is also the forum for ensuring that purchasers involve consumers in assessing local needs and monitoring the delivery of services.

Maternity Services Liaison Committees (MSLCs) were first defined by the Maternity Services Advisory Committee (MSAC). The MSAC was set up by the government in 1982 in response to the growing concern about the perinatal mortality rate. These compared unfavourably with other countries and demonstrated great differences around the country and between different social groups. The increasing consumer complaints about the maternity services and, in particular, the impersonal nature of the services led to the publication of *Maternity Care in Action*, a three volume report on antenatal, intrapartum and postnatal care. Part 1 (antenatal care) suggested that each health authority set up a maternity services liaison committee (DoH 1982).

This local committee brings together all professionals involved in maternity care with lay representatives of users of the services. Their purpose is two-fold: firstly to agree procedures and monitor their effectiveness, and secondly to ensure the best use of resources and professional skills available (DoH 1982). *Maternity Care in Action Part II* devotes a chapter to listing the functions of the MSLC (DoH 1984).

The role of the MSLC in the new NHS

Despite being 10 years old the role of the MSLC in helping to maintain standards in the provision of maternity care is as important today as it was then. A forum for discussion between the purchasers, user representatives and providers ensures that all sides have an active and equal say in service planning.

Despite the recognized importance of these local committees, no official guidance about the place of the MSLC in the new NHS has been published by the DoH (Lewinson 1994). The Winterton report on maternity care recommended that the role of the MSLC be strengthened so that they may channel the views of consumers into the planning and monitoring of maternity services (House of Commons Health Committee 1992). Although the very nature of the MSLC would make it an ideal format through which to monitor the maternity services, *Changing Childbirth*, regarded by many as the blueprint of the future maternity services, whilst advocating the formation of an MSLC in every health authority, fails to define clearly the future remit of MSLCs. This causes some concern to the National Childbirth Trust and the Community Health Council, the two organizations from which lay members on the MSLC tend to come (Lewinson 1994). Their disappointment will be shared by many who have served on successful MSLCs. *Changing Childbirth* recommends setting out action points and indicators of success. These could be used to guide the agenda for all MSLCs for the next 5 years. To date the role of the MSLC continues as before. In some Health Authorities the committees form a useful and constructive part in the planning of the local maternity services whilst in others the MSLC is merely given lip service and its role is regarded with little importance. In these areas the power continues to be maintained by the providers, with the user representative members having little say. Without guidance from the DoH, this very useful resource may continue to be used ineffectively.

Auditing the quality of service provision is very high on the NHS agenda. One of the roles of the MSLC for the future could be auditing the quality of maternity services. Maxwell (1984) argues that quality of care cannot be measured in a single dimension. Maxwell suggests six dimensions of health care quality which can be used to form the MSLC agenda together with monitoring the implementation of *Changing Childbirth*. Maxwell's set of quality criteria attempt to recognize the multifaceted nature of health care management (Maxwell 1984). The very nature of these components makes them interchangeable in any discussion about the organization of health care.

According to Maxwell each criterion must be viewed from two standpoints: that of the client and that of the professional. If the client is the main focus of the care process, surely greater weight should be given to the consumer's views. However, because many consumers may not be in the position of having a fully informed view about their needs, the six dimensions of quality of care can be used as a means of introducing an audit cycle. This requires assessing needs, planning care and ensuring that the service continues to meet the changing needs. This is but one means by which services can be audited, but it provides an ideal method by which the MSLC can be involved in monitoring maternity services.

INTERPROFESSIONAL WORKING

It is not only the views of the consumers that are essential if maternity services are to be accessible, appropriate and effective. The views of GPs, midwives, obstetricians and paediatrician all contribute to shaping the maternity services.

What part do midwives play in making decisions about the organization of maternity care? Reid (1993) believes that midwives, as the care providers closest to women, will have to be in the vanguard in ensuring that purchasers and providers implement the necessary changes to make maternity care women-centred.

An important part of this implementation is ensuring that staff at shop floor level are involved in planning, implementation and evaluation. Few midwives have come to grips with the new purchasing environment and the ways in which commissioning agencies specify the health services they want from provider maternity units (Farrow 1993). For many midwives the responsibility for this lies with the hospital financiers or business managers. Many midwives have little knowledge of what is laid out in the service specification for their unit and what the unit has signed up to provide. Ideally, service specifications should be used as a means to bring about change. These changes will have a direct impact on the midwives. Lack of knowledge of the process of purchasing care makes ownership of change very difficult. How can midwives plan care if they have no idea what the purchasers have demanded and what their employing provider units have agreed? A common example of this occurs when concern is shown because the unit activity levels (measured in number of deliveries) have dropped. The significance of this escapes midwives if they are unaware that most maternity care is still purchased as a block contract and that the level of activity agreed between purchasers and providers each year is based on the previous year's statistics. Understanding this concept means that their own involvement in collection of statistics becomes relevant rather than just being seen as yet more paperwork.

The role of midwives in assessing the needs of the local population and responding to these needs is extremely important. Midwives are in a unique position in their relationship with women and their families to become aware of and to ensure that services they provide meet local needs. Community midwifery services have an excellent opportunity to ask and learn from local women and the community at large. This in turn encourages women and their families to learn from midwives about the services available to them.

The provision of maternity care has become highly complex, involving the skills and time of a variety of professionals. The relationship between midwives and doctors, and obstetricians and GPs, is still burdened by role confusion and interprofessional rivalry in many units. Changing childbirth and the future of GP fundholding means that the future of many doctors in the provision of maternity care is far from certain, particularly with regard to the care of healthy pregnant women. Whether midwives are ready to take on the full responsibility of this group of women remains to be seen. However, it is clear that the current duplication of care is expensive and at times ineffective. It is questionable whether the current provision of maternity care meets Maxwell's test of effectiveness, efficiency and economy.

For too long, health care services have been organized to meet the needs of the workers and perpetuate the institution rather than planned and managed to serve the population (MacDonald 1991, Neuberger 1992). For many years this meant that maternity care was organized to meet the requirements of the service. However strong the need and desire to change practice, Ball *et al.* (1992) believe that at local level midwives, obstetricians and GPs still find it difficult to envisage and create change in the face of restricted resources, financial pressure, dearth of manpower and fears about implications of change. Commissioning agencies, however, are in the powerful position of bringing about change by ensuring that the care they purchase is effective and reflects the changes recommended in *Changing Childbirth*.

CONCLUSION

Alongside the battle between midwives and doctors as to who should take responsibility for the care of healthy pregnant women, another war is being fought – the battle to maintain the NHS and to ensure the survival of individual maternity units as they compete in the open market.

The future of midwifery depends on how we respond to the radical reforms in the NHS and the changing demand of the consumers of the service. It is clear that we cannot ignore the changing culture within the NHS. It is in the interests of the profession to ensure that midwives take an interest in how the needs of pregnant women are being assessed and ensure that the services they provide respond to these needs.

Perkins (1991) points out that it may never be possible to provide a perfect service since women's individual needs will develop and change with social and therapeutic change. However, it is reasonable to aim for a service that is constantly improving and responding to change. This, states Perkins, means that midwives (and purchasers) will need to look at familiar practices with fresh eyes, to see whether they continue to meet the needs of women and their families. It is all too easy for systems that have been in place for some time to become the status quo because they meet the midwives' need for security rather than the pregnant woman's need for care.

Competition is not a word that sits comfortably with those of us employed in the caring professions. It is intended to produce cheaper, high-quality products by driving out weaker providers. The question is whether competition and patient choice are compatible. In effect, they should be since the latter should govern the former.

In maternity care, midwives have an excellent opportunity to put the new internal market into practice. Not, as many believe, because midwifery care is cheaper (there is little evidence of this and it degrades the profession to work on this premise) but because midwives can provide the efficient and personalized maternity service that is central to the new NHS reforms.

Dillner (1991) believes that the future market leaders in pregnancy care will be those who can offer a package of community-based care with good continuity of care backed up by a good secondary care service. The battle between primary and secondary care-givers must be settled as the real victims of this rivalry are pregnant women. Struggles for territory and power are formidable barriers to effective care. Accepting the view of the Expert Maternity Group (DoH 1993b) that women with uncomplicated pregnancies should, if they wish, be able to book with a midwife as the lead professional for the entire episode of her pregnancy, including delivery in a general hospital, is an enormous cultural change. It is doubtful that midwives will ever work totally alone;

the need for obstetricians will always be there. Therefore close cooperation and collaboration is essential to ensure that appropriate and timely referrals are made. There can be little doubt that women will receive better quality of care from persons who are experienced in, and committed to, the principles of quality care as outlined in Maxwell's six dimensions of care and *Changing Childbirth*.

ACKNOWLEDGEMENT

My grateful thanks to Vicky Bailey for providing me with the idea for the desert island scenario on page 4.

REFERENCES

Ball, J. *et al*. (1992) *Who's Left Holding the Baby? An Organisational Framework for Making the Most of Midwifery Services*. Leeds: The Nuffield Institute for Health Service Studies.

Bowling, A. (1992) 'Assessing Health Needs and Measuring Patient Satisfaction', *Nursing Times*, Vol. 88, No. 31, July 29, pp. 31–3.

Bradshaw, G. and Bradshaw, P.L. (1994) Competition and efficiency in health care – the case of the British National Health Service, *Journal of Nursing Management* 2: 31–6.

Chalmers, I., Enkin, M. and Keirse, M.J.N.C. (eds) (1989) *Effective Care in Pregnancy and Childbirth*, Oxford: Oxford University Press.

Coates, P.M. (1994) Purchaser and provider contracts, In Chamberlain, G. and Patel, N. (1994) *The Future of the Maternity Services*, Chapter 17, London: RCOG Press.

Connah, B. and Pearson, R. (eds) (1991) *NHS Handbook*, 7th edn, Birmingham: National Association of Health Authorities and Trusts.

Department of Health (1982) *Maternity Care in Action Part I: Antenatal Care*, Crown copyright.

Department of Health (1984) *Maternity Care in Action Part II: Care During Childbirth*, Crown copyright.

Department of Health (1990) NHS and Community Care Act. London: HMSO.

Department of Health (1992) *The Patient's Charter*, London: HMSO.

Department of Health (1993a) *A Study of Midwife- and GP-led Maternity Units*, NHS Management Executive.

Department of Health (1993b) *Changing Childbirth Part 1: Report of the Expert Maternity Group*, London: HMSO.

Department of Health (1994) The Patient's Charter Maternity Services.

Dillner, L. (1991) Maternity services: the shaping of things to come, *British Medical Journal* **301:** 1198–2000.

Donaldson, R.J. and Donaldson, L.J. (1993) *Essential Public Health Medicine*, Dordrecht: Kluwer Academic Publishers.

Editorial (1992) *British Journal of General Practice*, October, pp. 401–5.

Farrow, S. (1993) 'Time to Look Through Those Specs', *MIDIRS Midwifery Digest*, Vol. 3, No. 2, June, pp. 225–6.

Gillam, S.J. (1992) 'Assessing the Health Care Needs of Populations – the General Practitioner's Contribution' (Editorial), *British Journal of General Practice*, October, pp. 404–5.

House of Commons Health Committee (Session 1991–92) (1992) *Second Report: Maternity Services*, London: HMSO.

Lewinson, H. (1994) *Maternity Services Liasion Committees. A Forum for Change. A Joint Briefing Paper from the Greater London Association of Community Health Councils and the National Childbirth Trust*, London: GLACHC.

MacDonald, J. (1991) Relative roles of midwife, general practitioner and obstetrician in the care of pregnant women in the next decade, *Contemporary Review of Obstetrics and Gynaecology* **3:** 201–4.

Martin, C. (1990) How do you count maternal satisfaction? A user-commissioned survey of maternity service. In Roberts, H. (ed.) *Women's Health Counts*, Chapter 6. London: Routledge.

Mason, V. (1989) Women's Experience of Maternity Care – A Survey Manual, London: HMSO.

Maternity Services: Government Response to the Second Report from the Health Committee (Session 1991–92) (1992) Cmnd 2018, London: HMSO.

Maxwell, R. (1984) Quality assessment in health, *British Medical Journal* **288:** 1470–2.

National Health Services Management Executive (1992) *Local Voices: the Views of Local People in Purchasing for Health*, London: Department of Health.

Neuberger, J. (1992) London after Tomlinson Community Health Services. *British Medical Journal*, **305:** 1486–8.

North East Thames Regional Health Authority (1992) *Advice to Purchasing Authorities on the Midwifery Component of Maternity Services*, London: North East Thames, November 1992.

Perkins, E.R. (1991) What do Women Want? Asking Consumers' Views. Midwives Chronicle and Nursing Notes, Vol. 104, No. 1247 (December), pp. 347–54.

Reid, T. (1993) 'Birth Pangs', *Nursing Times*, Vol. 27, No. 43, October 27, pp. 46–8.

Secretaries of State for Social Services, Wales, Northern Ireland and Scotland (1989a) *Working for Patients* (Cm 555), London: HMSO.

Secretaries of State for Social Services, Wales, Northern Ireland and Scotland (1989b) *Contracts for Services and the Role of District Health Authorities*, London: HMSO.

Stevens, A. and Gabbay, J. (1991) 'Needs Assessment Needs Assessment . . .', *Health Trends*, Vol. 23, No. 1, pp. 20–3.

Tyler, S. and Jenkins, R. (1994) Can GPs reach the high Cs? *Health Service Journal*, Vol. 104, No. 5387, p. 30.

Welsh Health Planning Forum (1991) Protocol for investment in health gain: maternal and early child health, Cardiff: Welsh Office NHS Directorate 1991.

Wilson, J. and McAnulty, L. (1991) *Resources for Practice*, London: Distance Learning Centre, South Bank Polytechnic.

2

Working from a Multiracial Perspective

Carol Baxter

Every woman has unique needs. In addition to those arising from her medical history these will derive from her particular ethnic, cultural, social and family background. The services provided should recognize the special characteristics of the population they are designed to serve. They should be attractive and accessible to all women . . .

(Department of Health 1993)

The above opening words of the Expert Maternity Group report, which sets out the key components of a woman-centred service, have brought the needs of ethnic minority women into sharper focus. Drawing from several secondary sources, including surveys of users' views across the country, this chapter explores black and ethnic minority women's experiences of maternity services and identifies prerequisites for an ethnically sensitive service. It also provides some quidelines as a starting point for midwives for improving personal practice.

MULTIRACIAL BRITAIN

In the 1991 Census almost 6% of the total British population described themselves as being black or from a minority ethnic group (Table 2.1) Although only 10 ethnic groups are identified, the 'other' categories in the census data are very important. Some of the main other ethnic groups that have been identified are: people of Asian origin from East Africa, Colombians, Chileans, Vietnamese, Filipinos, Travellers, Arabs, Central and Eastern Europeans, Italians, Portuguese, Moroccans, Greek Cypriots, Turkish Cypriots, Iranians, Yemeni,

Table 2.1   Ethnic composition of population in England
and Wales (Balarajan and Raleigh 1993)

	Number[a]	Percentage
White	46,936,500	94.1
Black Caribbean	499,000	1.0
Black African	205,400	0.4
Black – other	176,400	0.4
Indian	830,600	1.7
Pakistani	454,500	0.9
Bangladeshi	159,500	0.3
Chinese	147,300	0.3
Other Asian	193,100	0.4
Other	280,900	0.6
Total persons	49,883,200	

[a]Figures are rounded to nearest hundred.

Central Europeans and people of mixed ethnic and racial origin. Black and ethnic minority communities are not spread evenly across the country. Whilst in
some areas of the country there are few black and ethnic minority people, there
are significantly larger proportions in inner and outer areas of the three large
conurbations of London, Birmingham and Manchester, as well as in Leicester.
In some cities or boroughs such as Brent, Newham, Tower Hamlets, Hackney
and Ealing, black and ethnic minority people can make up over a third of the
local population. The multiracial nature of our society is therefore now well
recognized and no midwife in any part of the health services can go through her
career without having to think about the kind of care she offers to women from
this section of the population.

INEQUALITIES

Although the situation is changing, black and ethnic minority communities are
to a large extent still a young population. Maternity services are therefore one
of their main points of contact with the National Health Service (NHS).
However, studies have shown that black and ethnic minority women experience unequal access to maternity services and receive inadequate provisions of
these services to meet their needs (Pearson 1985). Through observation of use
of antenatal care a considerable amount of information about access to services
by women from this section of the population has been amassed. A study carried out in Leicester revealed that, as compared with 80% of non-Asians, only

64% of Asian mothers had over 5 months of supervised antenatal care (Clarke and Clayton 1983). A Bradford study showed similar patterns with 60% of Asian mothers having had less than 4 months antenatal care in comparison to 20% of non-Asian mothers (Lumb *et al.* 1981). Poor access to antenatal services by Afro-Caribbean women (Larbie 1985) and by travelling women (Save the Children Fund 1983) has also been recognized.

There is also substantial evidence that perinatal and infant mortality rates are also higher in babies whose mothers were born in the New Commonwealth and Pakistan (Amin and Oppenheim; Table 2.2). Poverty and deprivation, which black and ethnic minority communities are more likely to experience (Figure 2.1 and Table 2.3), are major contributors to this excess mortality. Maternity services, however, can have a considerable effect on the experiences and outcome of pregnancy.

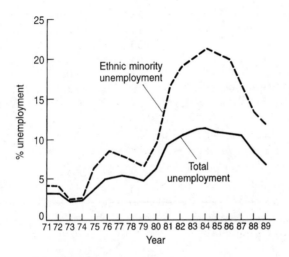

Figure 2.1 Racial disadvantage and the economic cycle: ethnic minority and total unemployment, 1971–89 (Amin and Oppenheim 1992)

INACCESSIBLE AND INAPPROPRIATE SERVICES

Good interpersonal relationships, communication and appropriate information are essential if women are to make informed choices. For black and ethnic minority women, however, difficulties in communication are more likely to arise owing to differences in language, experience, background and expectations between them and those providing services. Language barriers are therefore one of the most obvious factors that systematically jeopardize the standard

Table 2.2   Perinatal and infant deaths: number and rates per 1000 total births: by country of birth of mother in 1989 (England and Wales) (Amin and Oppenheim 1992)

Country of birth of mother	Perinatal deaths All ages		Infant deaths	
	Number	Rate	Number	Rate
All	5715	8.3	5701	8.3
United Kingdom	4928	8.1	4988	8.2
Irish Republic	54	8.2	65	9.9
Australia, Canada, New Zealand	24	8.6	23	8.3
New Commonwealth and Pakistan	544	10.9	466	9.4
New Commonwealth				
Bangladesh	56	10.9	30	5.9
India	91	10.2	81	9.2
East Africa	53	7.8	46	6.8
Rest of Africa	63	13.2	53	11.2
Caribbean Commonwealth	61	15.0	50	12.4
Mediterranean Commonwealth	16	6.3	21	8.4
Remainder of New Commonwealth	37	6.9	39	7.3
Pakistan	167	13.5	146	11.9
Remainder of Europe	67	7.0	64	6.7
Other	80	6.6	91	7.5

Table 2.3   Income and material and social deprivation by ethnic group in Islington in 1987 (Amin and Oppenheim 1992)

	Proportion with:		
	Net household income less than £3,900	High deprivation	
		Material	Social
	(%)	(%)	(%)
Afro-Caribbean	39	37	36
Asian	25	35	34
Irish	38	47	42
Cypriot	35	24	50
Other	32	39	34
White	29	33	34

of care they receive and which precludes them from stating their preferences. Whilst many women who have settled in Britain may be fluent in English for most everyday purposes such as work or shopping, they may not necessarily have acquired the rather specialized language needed for making sense of hospital systems, routines and diagnosis, medical procedures and treatment. Information about the types of maternity services available is not always available in the languages spoken by many ethnic minority women. Similarly, women do not always have access to information about how to prepare themselves for hospital and what to expect. For the same reasons preconceptual advice and antenatal classes are often felt to be inaccessible to women from this section of the population.

Language difficulties can also result in excessive waiting times for black and ethnic minority women. One study reported women having to sit around for hours virtually ignored whilst an interpreter is found or whilst the staff muster up the confidence or time to attempt some form of communication with them (Baxter 1993). Routine procedures such as history taking, the explanation of tests and test results, dietary or prenatal advice, admission and discharge home are aspects of care that pose particular problems. Some women often resort to bringing their own interpreters with them. As the following account demonstrates, reliance on relatives can often be unsatisfactory and can have serious consequences. A woman in labour ended up having an epidural which she categorically did not want but had no real choice or part in the decision. It transpired that when an epidural was suggested by the doctor, her mother-in-law, who was interpreting, did not herself understand what this meant and therefore conveyed the wrong information.

On the whole, because ethnic minority men and children are more likely to speak English than do women, they sometimes act as interpreters. Whilst this may appear on the surface to be a convenient arrangement, relatives are poor advocates because there may be conflicts of interest in terms of theirs and the woman's needs. Furthermore, instead of empowering the woman, their presence can be extremely embarrassing and degrading and often leaves the women with a lowered self-esteem.

Cultural and religious insensitivity

During pregnancy and childbirth, cultural insensitivity and misunderstandings can especially result in distress for women. An appreciation of, and a positive attitude towards, differences is thus essential in ensuring that professional practice is closely matched to individual cultural and religious needs. As the following explanation will demonstrate, care during the puerperium is particularly relevant in this respect. Although this has changed considerably, in Western

European cultures the first 6 weeks after delivery have traditionally been viewed as primarily a period of rest and recovery. This is especially important for many black and ethnic minority women who may be used to a total break from responsibility and who may therefore expect a lot of help in looking after themselves and their babies during this period. Some Muslim women may also wish to be confined to the home. Early mobilization following delivery, the move towards shorter hospital stay and arranging for the postnatal check at 6 weeks could therefore pose difficulty for some women who may find this practice confusing or even callous. Routine practices such as these should be viewed more flexibly and the reasons behind them not taken for granted but made explicit to all women, especially those from ethnic minority communities.

Personal and care routines often differ between cultural groups. It is indeed on the postnatal wards, where women have to rely on service providers for their most personal aspects of care, that black and ethic minority women seem to have most dissatisfaction. One general area of dissatisfaction for black and ethnic minority women is the practice on postnatal wards of a bath on the second post-operative day. This can be culturally offensive in several ways. Firstly, as discussed earlier, such early ambulation may not always be welcomed by women who may view this time as a period of total bed rest. Secondly, a wash may be preferred to a bath at this stage, this being based on the feeling that 'exposure' at such an early stage in the puerperium is dangerous to the mother's health. Thirdly, although it is standard practice in England, many people, especially those from ethnic minority communities, prefer to take showers: a bath is not necessarily viewed as hygienic.

To ensure respect for individuals and avoid damaging practices and confusion, it is essential that all women are able to follow the routines that they are used to.

Visiting arrangements can also be another problematic area for the women. In many communities, visiting relatives in hospitals is viewed as a social responsibility. It is not uncommon for family members, relatives and friends to visit in a group. This view can conflict with expectations of the staff on the wards for whom visiting is generally considered to be the domain primarily of the next of kin. This often leads to relatives being made to feel unwelcome.

Modesty is an important issue for all women. This takes on more importance for those women who prefer to adhere to religious teachings that stipulate clear moral codes around male/female relationships. Being seen by a male doctor, for example, can be extremely embarrassing and offensive for some women, as can having a male relative or husband as an interpreter – a point that has been mentioned earlier. In the latter situation this may also be embarrassing for the males concerned. In addition, hospital gowns, which are generally felt to be a fairly insignificant matter, can be of great importance for some women. Frequent concerns are that gowns do not cover the arms and the ankles or do not have secure fastenings – many women, especially if they are of the Muslim faith, find this extremely immodest. Muslim women wishing to secure more privacy on the wards often find their efforts thwarted:

As a Muslim I prefer to see more privacy on the ward. It is very difficult and embarrassing for me especially when I am feeding the baby. On one occasion I drew the curtains around my bed and the nurse came and drew them back. She said I was preventing the woman in the next bed from getting enough light.

Diet and dietary advice is an important part of care of pregnant and nursing women. To be effective this advice must be closely related to what people normally eat. In every culture (including traditional British culture) there are particular types of foods that pregnant and nursing mothers are either encouraged or discouraged from eating. Lack of the appropriate knowledge and training result in some midwives being unable to give appropriate advice or to develop a dialogue of their dietary needs.

EVERY WOMAN IS UNIQUE

As the previous discussion highlights, attention to cultural and religious needs is undoubtedly essential to individualized care. However, whilst recognizing the existence of group values and beliefs, it must be appreciated that people respond to their culture in singularly personal ways and adapt their lifestyle and behaviour to meet changing circumstances. A fine balance is necessary in which midwives are mindful of the need to treat all women as individuals and not merely as a member of an ethnic or cultural group. It is also essential to recognize that black and ethnic minority women fall into the category of being either British born, settled or new immigrants, the latter being increasingly less likely. Tailoring a care package on assumptions about what is required based solely on what has been read or heard from others is common practice. However, it is extremely unhelpful. Every effort should be made to get to know and respond to pregnant women as individuals and to find out from women what their individual preferences are. The reader is referred to Baxter (1988), which offers some suggestions for achieving this.

RACIAL DISCRIMINATION AND STEREOTYPING

Racism is a dynamic and complex force in society that takes many forms, most of which are covert and inherently part of the fundamental way in which services are planned and delivered. Institutional discrimination within the NHS is the more common and damning form of racism. This is where all people who come into contact with services are treated the same regardless of their differing needs. Known also as the colour-blind approach, black and ethnic minority people are treated in a way that assumes they are from the same racial, cultural and linguistic background as the rest of the white majority population. Hence, provision of services on the whole through the English medium only, inappropriate diet and dietary advice, and culturally insensitive personal care routines described above are all examples of this.

It has been argued that skin colour is the greatest single factor that governs society's attitudes to members of minority groups. Hence, people whose skin is visibly different from the white majority population are particularly vulnerable to racial discrimination (Pumphrey and Verma 1990). In addition to the institutional barriers, the behaviour of some individual practitioners towards black and ethnic minority women can also be based on negative stereotypes. Most midwives are often not consciously aware of the ideology of racism which shapes the way they respond to those for whom it is their responsibility to provide services. Indeed, most people in the caring professions would not deliberately withhold care or treat people differently on the basis of their colour. However, stereotyping is one way in which racism is perpetuated by individuals within services. Negative stereotyped views are still prevalent in our society and black and ethnic minority people continue to be seen and evaluated in this way. Larbie's study involving 30 young Afro-Caribbean women, for example, identified that the views held by some health care workers made these women feel isolated and alienated. One woman had this to say:

This sister said to me, 'You black people have too many babies.' As far as I was concerned, I wasn't 'you black people', I was me. You don't forget something like that. . . . She was supposed to be caring for me.

(Larbie 1985)

Another study examining the stereotypes of women of South Asian descent, conducted by the University of Wales in Cardiff (Bowler 1993), identified that these women were particularly vulnerable to negative typification by midwives. The midwives' stereotypes contained four main themes: the difficulty of communicating with the women (in cases where this was not so); the women's lack of compliance with care and abuse of the service; their tendency to make a fuss about nothing; and their lack of normal maternal instinct. Midwives used such stereotypes to help them make judgements about the kinds of care different women want, need and deserve. This can in turn impact on the behaviour of individual midwives. Subsequently women from black and ethnic minority communities sometimes feel that they are treated with disrespect and unfavourably when using maternity services (Baxter 1993).

In acknowledging the pervasiveness of this form of racial discrimination, the Chief Medical Officer's Report (1991) states that 'The NHS must . . . and take positive steps to eliminate the effects of racial disadvantage and discrimination'. It is important to bear in mind that services and thus the staff who deliver them do not have complete discretion in this area but are obliged to observe the 1976 Race Relations Act. Under this act racial discrimination and segregation on grounds of colour, race or nationality, including citizenship or national origin, is unlawful. Appendix 2 provides details of the provisions of the Act. The Commission of Racial Equality (1994) has also produced the Race Relations Code of Practice in Maternity Services. This is aimed at helping all those who plan and deliver maternity services to be more responsive to the needs of their multiracial clientelle.

ETHNICALLY SENSITIVE SERVICES

The needs of black and ethnic minority women are often viewed as special when in fact they are not dramatically different from those of their white counterparts. All pregnant women have the right to a good standard of care. This comprises the availability of preconceptual advice and care, a choice of female doctors if preferred, sensitive communication from health professionals and appropriate diet while in hospital.

In summarizing the views expressed by black and ethnic minority pregnant women, several issues can be identified as prerequisites for developing services that are more accessible and appropriate to their needs. The following provides a summary of these:

- Information about services should be available in appropriate languages and should, in content and illustration, reflect a multiracial population.
- The additional use of videos and language cassettes should also be explored for both preconceptual and parentcraft advice.
- English for pregnancy classes should be considered as an additional way of ensuring information is understood, enabling women to understand services, the choices available and to ask questions.
- Information about important areas such as the signs of labour and practical information about how to telephone the hospital or midwife and what to take to the hospital may need to be repeated several times.
- The timing, siting and publicizing of antenatal classes should be planned in consideration of the needs of the women. Bilingual workers will need to

be available at the classes and to accompany the women on visits to the maternity units.

- There should be in-service development and training of midwives and other staff in the unit to address the language and cultural issues, interpersonal communication, religious and cultural practices and beliefs surrounding childbirth and the importance of asking women their preferences.
- There should be opportunities in training for staff to raise and discuss issues surrounding race and ethnicity and to examine their own attitudes towards members of minority groups.
- Staff responsible for history-taking should be trained in interviewing skills and the importance of taking time.
- There should be recruitment of student midwives from black and ethnic minority communities and especially those who are bilingual.

BLACK AND ETHNIC MINORITY STAFF

Midwives from black and ethnic minority communities, especially those from similar cultural backgrounds, who speak the language of their clients have an important role to play in delivering ethnically sensitive maternity services. However, this should not be automatically assumed to be so. Black and ethnic minority midwives are subjected to the same training and professional norms, policies and role models as their white colleagues. Furthermore, there are still insufficient midwives from this section of the population, many find that their particular perspectives, experiences and skills are undervalued and too few are in a position to make decisions within services.

The employment of bilingual workers in the NHS specifically to improve access to services for patients who speak little or no English, or those whose preferred language is other than English, has developed slowly over the past decade. These workers are employed under several different job titles, with a number of differing roles. Interpreters provide word for word interpretation between patients/clients and health professionals. In addition to interpreting, linkworkers have an additional role of providing information about available services and of acting as a bridge between the patient/client and health professional and ensuring that the patient is fully informed of the available options. Advocates have the additional role of advocacy, which includes acting on behalf of the patient/client to ensure that their preferences for treatment and services are achieved.

Whilst it is recognized that there is no absolute blueprint for a bilingual service and that areas will need to address local needs, the following example of initiatives within one Health District has positive features.

Hackney Community Health Council (CHC) pioneered a bilingual workers scheme in Britain. In 1980, borrowing from the ideas and ways of working from community projects in the Third World and from patient advocacy schemes in the USA, it funded the Multi-ethnic Women's Health Project.[1]

Hackney has a rich ethnic population mix which is constantly changing. Besides the indigenous cockneys the most established communities are the Jewish, African/Caribbean and more recently Turkish and Kurdish people. There is also a diverse Asian population from Uganda, Kenya, Bangladesh, Pakistan and India and a refugee population with people most recently coming from Vietnam, Somalia, Eritrea, Iraq and former Yugoslavia.

The aim of the scheme is to:

- improve access to the health service for non-English speaking women during pregnancy, childbirth and the postnatal period;
- advise the health authority on policy and practice with regard to the needs of non-English speaking women;
- help and encourage health service staff to provide a service to this high-risk group.

In this scheme the emphasis of training for advocates is on reinforcing the worker's existing knowledge and commitment, supplementing it on demand and helping them to develop new skills or knowledge as appropriate. Half a day per week is allocated to support and skill development and discussion of on-going problems. One of the District's specialists, for example, does occasional sessions on clinical care. The advocates have also had training sessions on counselling skills. The midwifery tutor ran six sessions on the basics of midwifery. The invitation to this session was extended to community workers who came into contact with pregnant women. An important area in training is the emphasis on joint training sessions with midwives and other service deliverers to facilitate mutual understanding of, and respect for, roles and responsibilities.

There are currently six advocates delivering language support services in Bengali, Urdu/Gujerati, Punjabi/Hindi, Turkish, Vietnamese, Chinese and Somali/Arabic. The advocates attend all the antenatal clinics within the hospital. They work closely with both the pregnant women and the staff. In the clinic this includes conducting the booking interview, filling in the booking forms and entering it on the computer. They take the women through the system, accompanying them into the consultation with the doctors to ensure that the women understand what is happening and that the staff have all the relevant information about them. During these visits the advocates ensure that the woman has received the appropriate advice on diet, has understood the various tests, knows what to do if she has a problem and what to do when she goes into labour. If necessary they support the women through scans, amniocentesis, abortion, miscarriage and family crisis. The advocates also visit the wards daily, sometimes staying with the women during delivery. They deal with problems with food, make sure the mother has had help with breast feeding, knows how to sterilize bottles and has the family planning advice she wants. After the women are discharged home they visit them at home at least once and more often if necessary.

As their job title implies, advocacy is a major feature of the worker's role; this occurs at two levels. Firstly, at the level of the individual patient, the advocate finds out information from the hospital for the patient, and helps the patient understand the purpose and methods of investigations, treatments and helps the patient to make their own wishes known to the hospital. A second and more demanding level is where the advocate's task is to bring to the attention of the relevant bodies anything in their policies and practices that is contrary to the patient's interest. The advocate's role is therefore one that continually challenges the deep-rooted belief held within the medical profession that the doctor is always right. They also challenge racism whether it is intentional or not and help seek solutions to more acceptable ways of working.

Recent studies carried out within Hackney also provide evidence of the impact of bilingual services on clinical outcome. A retrospective study compared 1,000 non-English speaking women delivering at the Mother's Hospital Hackney in 1986, who had been accompanied by an advocate, with women delivering at the same hospital in 1979 and at a reference hospital (Whipps Cross). Its findings showed significant differences between the groups in three outcomes: antenatal length of stay, induction, and mode of delivery. Although these changes cannot be directly attributed to bilingual workers, it was considered reasonable to deduce that improved communication could have influenced clinical practice. The findings suggest that health advocacy may offer a mechanism to address some of the adverse obstetric outcomes observed in ethnic minorities. The study concluded that if a bilingual health advocacy scheme can reduce interventions while increasing patient satisfaction, it is a good investment (Parsons and Day 1992). This view is also reflected in the recent report of the Department of Health Expert Maternity Group which states that:

> *When a maternity unit is providing services to significant numbers of women who are unable to communicate in English, it is essential that providers should develop linkworker and advocacy schemes. Linkworkers and advocates should not be seen as optional extras to the service. They should be fully integrated into the maternity care team . . .*

> (Department of Health 1993)

Another more recent innovation in Hackney is the use of a minority language word processing package, which includes keyboard templates for 10 languages most commonly used by pregnant women seen in Homerton Hospital in Hackney. They will translate and edit maternity leaflets covering a wide range of subjects including pain relief in labour, complications of labour, Caesarean section, breast and bottle feeding, health eating, family planning and HIV. The leaflets are being made available in GP surgeries, antenatal classes, clinics and on the delivery suites when women are admitted to labour.

INDIVIDUAL ACTION

The action areas identified above relate to required changes in organizational practice and are outside the powers of the individual midwife. However, some personal action is also required to bring about changes in individual attitudes, as is some personal adjustment in ways of working. It is essential for midwives not to become paralysed by the scale of the task – awareness and concern on its own will not help to improve professional competence.

Whilst acquiring cultural information can be beneficial, a more appropriate starting point is to reflect on personal attitudes and beliefs. For many white people brought up in a predominantly white environment, prejudices – often based on ignorance and self-interest – can run very deep. It can often be difficult to be honest about such feelings and beliefs: few like to admit that they hold, or have held, racist attitudes, or give credence to racist stereotypes. However, negative images of black people have been very persistent and are still evident in many parts of the health service. These have negative effects and interfere with the development of positive, open relationships between midwives and the women for whom they provide services. However, the habit of being reflective – making explicit personal values, making a genuine attempt to understand and acknowledge the experiences of black and ethnic minority people, challenging racial discrimination (intentional or otherwise) where it occurs and developing ways of responding to black and ethnic minority people that value their cultures; will enhance professional competence.

Midwives who wish to evaluate their own attitudes, knowledge and practical skills will need to think about the following:

- What means are available to you to learn about the nature of racism and how it affects your work practice?
- Is your relationship with black and ethnic minority women influenced by commonly held stereotypes?
- What skills have you developed to find out about the cultural and religious needs of individual pregnant women?

- What have you done to find out what your hospital's or authority's policies are on equal opportunities and race relations?
- Do you know what facilities there are to assist in the care of ethnic minority women in your hospital and in the community?

SUMMARY AND CONCLUSION

Poor access to maternity services and worse birth outcomes by black and ethnic minority women is now well recognized. Women from this section of the population are also often dissatisfied with the quality of services they receive. Poor socioeconomic status and language and communication difficulties are among the reasons for these inequalities. Good communication is also prevented when health workers have negative attitudes towards black and ethnic minority women, whether these attitudes are conscious or not. This interferes with the development of positive, open relationships between midwives and women from this section of the population.

Like most other large bureaucratic organizations the NHS has tended to develop an inflexible structure and many of its services (including those aimed at pregnant women) are specially geared to the needs of the dominant culture.

The employment of patient advocates is viewed as important in improving maternity services to black and ethnic minority women. The main focus is on facilitating changes in the service so that it is delivered from a perspective that takes account of diversity in cultural and religious beliefs and challenging racial discrimination in services. Health Authorities and Provider Units are at different stages of development in their response to the need for ethnically sensitive services. Indeed, there are increasing numbers of examples of good practice across the country.

Several organizational and personal actions that are prerequisites of any strategy to improve services to women from this section of the population have been identified which, although they require sustained and systematic effort, are within grasp.

NOTE

1. Further information about the Hackney Multi-ethnic Women's Project is available from: Hafice Ece, Coordinator, The Multi-ethnic Women's Project, City and Hackney Community Health Council, 210 Kingsland Road, London E2 8EB, UK.

REFERENCES

Amin, K. and Oppenheim, C. (1992) *Poverty in Black and White: Deprivation and Ethnic Minorities.* London: Child Poverty Action Group with the Runnymede Trust.

Balarajan, R. and Raleigh, V. (1993) *Ethnicity and Health: A Guide for the NHS,* London: Department of Health.

Baxter, C. (1988) 'Culture Shock', *Nursing Times,* January 13, Vol. 84, No. 2.

Baxter, C. (1993) *The Communication Needs of Black and Ethnic Minority Pregnant Women in Salford.* Unpublished Report available from Nick Walbank, Purchasing Department, Salford Health Authority.

Bowler, I. (1993) 'They're not the same as us. Midwives Stereotypes of South Asian Descent Maternity Patients', *Sociology of Health and Illness,* Vol. 15, No. 2.

Calman, K.C. (1992) On the state of Public Health 1991: The Annual Report of the Chief Medical Officer of the Department of Health for the year 1991. London: HMSO.

Clarke, M. and Clayton, D. (1983) Quality of obstetric care provided for Asian immigrants in Leicestershire, *British Medical Journal* **280:** 621–3.

Commission of Racial Equality (1994) *Race Relations Code of Practice in Maternity Services: For the Elimination of Racial Discrimination and the Promotion of Equal Opportunities,* London: Commission of Racial Equality.

Department of Health (1993) *Changing Childbirth. Part 1: Report of the Expert Maternity Group,* London: HMSO.

Larbie, J. (1985) Black women and maternity services. In *Training in Health and Race,* National Extension College, London.

Lumb, K.M., Longden, P.J. and Lealman, G.T. (1981) A comparative review of Asian and British born maternity patients in Bradford, *Journal of Epidemiology and Community Health* **35:** 106–9.

Parsons, L. and Day, S. (1992) Improving obstetric outcomes in ethnic minorities: an evaluation of health advocacy in Hackney, *Journal of Public Health Medicine* **14:** 183–91.

Pearson M. (1985) *Racial Equality and Good Practice in Maternity Care,* Health Education Council and National Extension College.

Pumphrey, P.D. and Verma, G.K. (eds) (1990) *Race Relations in Urban Education,* Hampshire: Falmer Press.

Save the Children Fund (1983) *The Health of Traveller Mothers and Children in East Anglia,* London: Save the Children Fund.

3

An Interprofessional Approach to Care: Lessons from General Practice

Chris Ford and Steve Iliffe

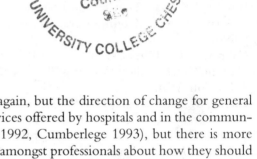

SCHOOL OF NURSING
Library
01033840
16 AUG 1999
Counter
Site
UNIVERSITY COLLEGE CHESTER

Maternity care is changing, once again, but the direction of change for general practitioners (GPs) is unclear. Services offered by hospitals and in the community are under review (Winterton 1992, Cumberlege 1993), but there is more certainty amongst politicians than amongst professionals about how they should develop. Perhaps the variety of interest groups with different perspectives on maternity care, coupled with the uncertainties and instability created by the National Health Service (NHS) 'reforms', mean that no clear programme for change can emerge, at least in the short term.

Over the last 15 years, obstetric practices that have become established despite a lack of supporting scientific evidence are being challenged by vocal women (Oakley 1979), by midwifery organizations (Kitzinger 1988) and by members of the medical profession itself (Zander and Chamberlain 1984, Campbell and Macfarlane 1987). The assumption that there is no alternative to hospital-based maternity care remains contested, within medicine itself (Marsh 1982). Relationships between professionals are being reviewed with the role of the GP in community obstetrics being questioned, whilst some – but not all – midwives are seeking greater professional autonomy.

A new generation of healthy, articulate and educated women are seeking a more personal and less technical approach to pregnancy and birth. Organizations such as the Association for Improvement in Maternity Services (AIMS) and the National Childbirth Trust (NCT) have focused attention on the quality of maternity care and reopened debate on the issue of safety in pregnancy and labour. Safety, which was seen by most obstetricians as the paramount consideration when planning maternity care in the early years of the NHS, has been joined by satisfaction and the psychological well-being of the mother as important outcomes in the perception of many women, and an increasing number of professionals. Economic considerations are also entering the picture, as successive governments try to cut health care costs by finding cheaper ways of providing services whilst meeting professional demands for less arduous work schedules.

All change is difficult for those caught up in it. The current transformation in health care exposes the strengths and weaknesses of professional attitudes and work styles, and poses threats to the quality of services, but it also creates opportunities for developing better maternity care based on greater public involvement and enhanced collaboration between professionals. In this chapter we will discuss the potential for community-based multidisciplinary maternity care, the impact it could have on specialist maternity services and the ways in which it could be developed.

For us the best way to describe the problems of public involvement and professional education is to address the issue that has been debated so much in the 1980s, and which has demonstrated the gulf between professional and public perception of good practice, as well as the differences between obstetrics and midwifery. Where should babies be born?

THE PLACE OF BIRTH

At the moment women can give birth with professional support in three places: a consultant-led hospital maternity unit; a GP maternity unit (in or separate from a District General hospital); or in their own home. The great majority of women opt for a hospital birth, in a consultant-led unit. Limited choice may account for the predominance of the hospitals, because the number of GP units has diminished and, until very recently, home birth has been opposed actively by the great majority of obstetricians. However, opportunity is not the only explanation, for even an optimistic prediction of the demand for home births suggested that only one in four women would make this choice (Huntingford 1980). Birth in hospital is seen as safe, and many pregnant women value the reduction of risk to themselves and their babies that hospital maternity units seem to represent.

Hospital maternity units

The issue of safety in pregnancy and labour is not as straightforward as is sometimes portrayed by hospital obstetricians. The application of modern obstetric technology may result in inappropriate interventions in the pregnancy or labour to the low-risk mother, putting the mother and baby at risk from new and different problems as well as undermining the clinical confidence of both midwives and junior doctors (Tew 1985). Low-risk women giving birth in GP units have shown less intervention, less episiotomies and greater patient satisfaction (Klein *et al.* 1993). Experience from Holland, where care by the midwife and delivery at home or in a midwife-led unit is seen as the first option, shows satisfaction, low perinatal mortality rates and low rates of instrumental delivery (Van Alten *et al.* 1989).

The widespread availability and further development of obstetric technology can be both beneficial and hazardous. Any technology that assists a women to give birth to a well baby is desirable, but the danger in the current repertoire of labour induction, fetal monitoring and advanced pain relief lies both in its misuse by poorly trained staff working pathologically long hours under pressure, and in its capacity to deskill clinicians. Obstetrics is less scientific than we are led to believe, and there are great variations in clinical judgement between experienced obstetricians. Fetal monitoring during labour has become almost an obligation in hospital obstetrics, but it is an extremely limited method for assessing fetal health (Nielson 1993). Routine induction of labour at term has become routine practice in some maternity units, although ultrasound scanning shows that half or more of 'post-term' pregnancies are actually less than 40 weeks gestation. There appears to be no 'right time' to induce labour after term, and there is no evidence available with which to develop a rational policy (Cardozo 1993).

A retrospective audit by senior clinicians of emergency Caesarean sections performed over a 15-year period at St James' Hospital, Leeds, suggested that up to 30% of the operations were unnecessary (Barrett *et al.* 1990). Most of these emergency Caesarean sections were performed for fetal distress, a diagnosis that relies on the output of fetal monitors or on the results of fetal blood sampling. Relatively inexperienced obstetricians-in-training form the bulk of the labour ward medical workforce, especially outside the normal working day. Some may be in their first Senior House Officer (SHO) post, with very little experience of normal labour and birth, but with a high level of anxiety that accentuates their reliance on medical authority and limits their absorption of midwife experience. These doctors, and the Registrars and Senior Registrars who supervise them, may overestimate the accuracy of cardiotocograph tracings, overvalue the significance of fetal blood acidity and over-ride the assessments of experienced midwives, leading to an 'emergency' that might have been avoided. In the Leeds study the audit also revealed that the auditors themselves disagreed with each other often, and were inconsistent in their personal judgements in 25% of cases when asked to review the same births some time later. We can only speculate on the impact these inconsistencies have on working relationships between midwives and doctors, but our experience and observations give us the impression that arbitrary decisions imposed with medical authority undermine midwives' confidence, are corrosive of teamwork and do not enhance collaboration.

The deaths of mothers and babies are rare enough now, but the fear of them pervades obstetric practice, with the result that small probabilities are over-weighted and disasters loom larger psychologically in clinical decision-making than they do in an objective assessment of risk (Balla *et al.* 1989). Fear of an obstetric disaster is a potent force for adopting a rigid, protocol-driven approach to labour, and a depersonalizing attitude towards the woman in labour. Raphael-Leff (1991) describes the impact of staff anxiety on maternity ward activities very well. Maternity ward staff may tend to concentrate on task-oriented work, rather than on 'whole patient' treatment, and may depersonalize pregnant women to reinforce the view that all pregnant women are the same (and therefore suitable subjects for a protocol-driven approach to labour). Staff may see themselves as equally interchangeable, and come and go accordingly. Ritualization of treatment reduces uncertainty and the need for personal initiative and decision-making, and technology acts as an excellent prop for such standardized rituals. In practice, of course, this interchangeability is limited, and different staff may express very different views whilst perceiving themselves as units in a consistent team.

Great efforts have been applied within midwifery, and to a lesser extent in obstetrics, to avoid the use of these defence mechanisms and to make maternity care centre upon the pregnant woman. Like all anxiety-avoidance mechanisms, they are hard to change. For example, 20% of doctors and midwives interviewed in a recent study in Oxfordshire said that they would continue weighing pregnant women routinely even if prospective trials showed that this activity had no impact on outcome (Dawes *et al.* 1992). Community staff have the advantage of always being vulnerable both to criticism and to emotional involvement because of their one-to-one relationships with pregnant women in their own homes, and can learn how to deal with their vulnerability in ways that are less depersonalizing than those adopted in the factory environment of the hospital. Transfer of these techniques from community services to the maternity wards of hospitals may help the processes of change currently underway in hospital maternity units.

General practitioner units

There is a variety of ways in which community midwives and GPs work together in 'GP maternity units'. Some units are free-standing, staffed by midwives with the GP on call, and others are in District General hospitals with instant access to specialist obstetricians and obstetric technology. Free-standing units have decreased in number, and conventional obstetric wisdom perceives their isolation from specialist units as unsafe. The quality of GP obstetrics has been criticized frequently by hospital specialists, with recent debate becoming heated. A paper reviewing the outcome of GP obstetrics in Bradford reported high perinatal mortality and stillbirth rates, and called for tighter controls over the experience of doctors participating in a fully integrated system of obstetric care (Bryce *et al.* 1990). The acrimonious correspondence that followed publication of this research revealed the depth of antagonism between specialists and GPs in Bradford, as well as airing many criticisms of the design, conduct and presentation of a report that appeared to contain many fallacies and false conclusions (Johnson 1990).

A similarly flawed paper on perinatal mortality rates in isolated GP maternity units around Bath prompted a similar debate about hasty and tendentious conclusions drawn from inadequate information (Sangala *et al.* 1990). The adversarial nature of the debate obscured the concluding comments in the initial report, which anticipated the benefits of an extra consultant obstetrician in the Bath area and so hinted at the relative lack of specialist medical expertise in the local maternity services. An extra consultant might facilitate collaboration between disciplines and across the hospital–community interface, but this work has been made all the harder by the polemical use of poorly understood data.

In the early 1980s 25% of GPs were involved in intra-partum care (Marsh 1985). Now the proportion is less than 10% and falling (Bull 1988) and some question whether there is a future for general practice obstetrics at all (Jewell and Smith 1990). Perhaps predictably, a review of the contribution of GPs to hospital intra-partum care throughout England and Wales received less publicity than the Bradford and Bath reports, although its findings suggested a significant decline in GP involvement (Smith and Jewell 1991).

The reviewers found that the number of isolated GP maternity units had declined rapidly, and all births in GP units accounted for only 5.9% of total births. GPs tended to be less involved in clinical reviews and the policy-making process when working alongside consultant-led units. The authors concluded: 'We may be witnessing not only the terminal decline of general practitioner intra-partum care but also the start of a long process in which general practitioners are excluded from having any say in obstetric care' (Smith and Jewell 1991).

This pessimism is understandable, but it may also be a reflection of past power relationships. If the market culture pervades health care, the balance of power may well shift away from hospital-based obstetrics and more towards community-based midwifery, if only because there are potential cost savings and quality gains in a midwife-led service. GPs will be able to make a real, if modest, contribution to this shift in emphasis if they can adopt a supportive role towards community midwives and also provide information about service quality to purchasers. We will discuss these possibilities in more depth later in this chapter.

Home birth

Birth at home used to be commonplace until the late 1950s and birth in hospital was only indicated if an adverse history or problems in the current pregnancy warranted specialist care. Figure 3.1 shows a letter from a hospital obstetrician to a GP, found in the medical records of one patient. It shows how hospital birth required specific 'indications' at a time when hospital maternity units were smaller than now. Hospital-based maternity services expanded at the same time as women's health improved and the perinatal mortality fell. The improvement in outcomes was attributed (uncritically, in our view) to the impact of specialist care in hospital maternity units, and births at home decreased from 50% of all births in 1954 to 1% in 1980, after which the rate has remained static (Loudon 1990).

Birth in hospital has become the norm in Britain (and in the USA) but not everywhere in the industrialized world. In Holland, birth at home remains normal, and 43% of women have their babies under the care of independent midwives with no evidence of worse outcomes for mother or baby as a consequence (Treffers *et al.* 1990). In the UK birth at home is possible, even in deprived inner-city areas, although it remains an option chosen mainly by the most educated (Ford *et al.* 1991). The experience of the authors in providing GP obstetric support for women having their babies at home over the last 15 years is unusual, but not unique, and similar provision exists in East and South London and Sheffield. Figure 3.2 shows the outcomes for women opting for home births in one inner London practice between 1979 and 1989, and demonstrates how safe home birth can be for a self-selected group of pregnant women with good community midwife teams.

The necessary ingredients for this level of GP contribution to community maternity care seem to be supportive colleagues, working in a large practice (six doctors) with relatively low list sizes (1980 patients per doctor) and a relatively low consultation rate (3.2 consultations/year), and sympathetic hospital consultants. Even with these favourable background circumstances, cooperation across professions can be difficult. In this London area there are three different midwife teams, each related to a different maternity unit, and each working in a different way. Working patterns change as staff change, and our relationships with these teams have to be re-made to allow collaboration with new personalities and attitudes.

If working relationships are not reviewed and developed explicitly and regularly, problems arise. For example, a new midwife on one team tells the GP

PADDINGTON GROUP HOSPITAL MANAGEMENT COMMITTEE

PADDINGTON GENERAL HOSPITAL

HOSPITAL SECRETARY   HARROW ROAD,   TELEPHONE:
D.M. DOIG. B.A., A.H.A.   LONDON, W.9.   CUNNINGHAM 4884

REH/KF   12th December, 1963.

Dear Dr. ███████

    re Mary ███████ age 26 years
████████████████████████████████████

    Thank you for your letter about this patient, who is 16 weeks pregnant.

    There are no social or medical grounds for booking her for hospital confinement.

    I have referred her back to you to arrange for home confinement.

    Yours sincerely,

Figure 3.1   A letter from a hospital obstetrician to a GP.

on–call for obstetrics about a woman in labour at home, only when a problem has arisen and has been resolved, during a prolonged second stage of labour. The GP is at some distance from the woman's home, and involves another doctor who is nearer. The crisis is over when the GP arrives, and so is the labour. At first glance mother and baby seem well, but the midwife is visibly relieved at the outcome and the mother has had an anxious hour when she sensed that something was

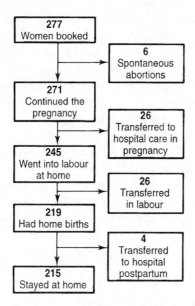

Figure 3.2 Outcome of pregnancy in women booked for home birth during 1977–89.

going wrong, but could do nothing about it. Things do not go well in the next few days. A tear sutured within an hour of the birth breaks down in 2 days. The baby is jittery and a problem to feed, although this resolves in a few days. Earlier contact would have put the on-call doctor in a better position to reach the home, and even if the GP's presence would not have altered the conduct of the second stage, at least it might have diminished the anxiety of both parties.

The central professional in a home birth is the community midwife, and the GP is one of her supports. In the author's experience, midwives undertaking home births must feel competent in their skills and confident about their medical back-up. This back-up includes the GP who knows the pregnant woman, the local midwifery team and the local maternity unit. Midwives too are mainly trained in the hospital setting, and may be used to having equipment only available in hospital around them. Many of the midwives who have had years of experience of supporting pregnant women through to birth in the community are retiring and their skills and confidence are being lost.

Easy access to all the facilities of the labour ward, including obstetricians who understand and value what is happening in the community, is essential. Here the attitude of consultants is crucial, for they can influence the behaviour of junior staff in important ways. A woman in labour transferring from home to hospital in the middle of the night gains little from a pompous registrar who is openly critical of the community midwife or the woman herself, and given the anxieties created by pregnancy and birth and the sometimes pathological mood of the labour ward, frequent discussion of how to deal with different perceptions of risk and safety may be an important task of the GP obstetrician.

Where home birth is accepted in principle, obstacles may be created in practice. Guidelines for deciding which women can safely have their babies at home may be rigid and inflexible, perhaps excluding women in their first pregnancy or women over an arbitrary age from the option of a 'sanctioned' home birth, even though these exclusion criteria may no longer be rational. The Dutch approach to listing the indications for specialist involvement through pregnancy and labour may be a better approach (Oppenheim 1993). Community midwives may feel deskilled by their long-standing relegation to antenatal and postnatal care, and be anxious about their competence and the mother's safety. These are real problems that cannot be wished away, but they can be changed given commitment, time and mutual tolerance between professionals, and also between pregnant women and those working in the maternity services.

BEFORE AND AFTER BIRTH

It is possible to get passionate about the place and manner of birth, but what about pregnancy? Routine antenatal was started between the First and Second World Wars when much less was known about the physiology and psychology of pregnancy (Marsh 1991). Women or their babies frequently died in pregnancy or labour and anything that prevented this could only be seen as a good thing. Regimented measuring of certain physiological parameters such as weight, blood pressure and urinary protein could identify some abnormal pregnancies, and obstetric science focused on treating these abnormalities and minimizing risk to mother and baby (Hall 1993). Standardized and ritualistic antenatal care became routine without its scientific validity being demonstrated, simply because it made both intellectual and emotional sense in the then current climate of knowledge, and the prevailing anxiety about the hazards of pregnancy and birth.

We can now judge antenatal routines more critically, and see that activities such as routine weighing fail to predict the onset of an important pregnancy hazard, pre-eclampsia (Dawes *et al.* 1992). A reduced programme of antenatal care does not compromise early detection of correctable abnormalities and does allow redeployment of midwife and doctor time (Hall *et al.* 1980). The same rigidly structured approach to postnatal care, together with the pressure of work on postnatal wards, contributes to the current low rates of breast feeding, with staff attitudes so ambivalent that a campaign for a 'baby friendly hospital' is a serious proposition (Waterston and Davies 1993).

What should these redeployed doctors and midwives do? And what is the emotional climate that will shape professional activity in maternity care in the next decades? Raphael-Leff's description of different attitudes to pregnancy, birth and parenthood may be a good guide to the new orientation needed in community-based maternity care (Raphael-Leff 1991). She points to two extreme and polarized responses to pregnancy, each of which has implications for the conduct of pregnancy, the nature of the birth and subsequent parental behaviour. 'Facilitators' perceive pregnancy as the high point of their womanhood, become absorbed in it and want birth to be 'natural'. 'Regulators' experience pregnancy as an irritating stage on the way to having a baby, want to keep the process of pregnancy under control, and seek a civilized birth. Most pregnant women have features of both types, but tend to one or other pole of this spectrum in each pregnancy, although they may change poles with subsequent pregnancies.

A GP or an experienced community midwife with previous knowledge of the women, other children, the rest of the family and the community can provide continuity of care probably more than any other professional, precisely because they observe and learn to respond to variations in mood, attitude and belief along the 'facilitator–regulator' spectrum. Continuity of care matters because it increases the effectiveness of communication between the pregnant woman and her professional helpers, and this in turn increases the success of intervention (should any be needed) and also improves maternal satisfaction with the service (Smith 1990).

Midwives and GPs may not put their knowledge into these terms, or even express it explicitly, but they certainly use it. This knowledge can be shared amongst professionals working in the same community, which explains why having a small group of midwives can improve care for women, and why schemes such as the 'Know your midwife project' have shown greater women satisfaction, less use of analgesia in labour and less need for instrumental deliveries (Flint et al. 1989). GPs working with local community midwives can share that continuity and family knowledge.

Deleting ritualistic and unnecessary practices from antenatal and postnatal care does not mean abandoning all care, simply rationalizing it. There is now little doubt that most antenatal care can best be done in the community by small teams of midwives with GPs in a supportive role as both professionals with knowledge of their patients and doctors with some level of obstetric expertise (Street et al. 1991), although sometimes women will choose their GP as the key professional.

THE NEED FOR CHANGE

We have outlined the differences in perception between the public, obstetricians, midwives and GPs and the rigid attitudes and forms of organization that can arise from such differences. Can perceptions be shared, and can organization become flexible, so that maternity services can meet the needs and expectations of women in the 21st century? In particular, can professionals learn to collaborate?

In our view the desire for more collaborative and less dysfunctional styles of working is strong, and many of the efforts at reorganizing local services prefigure more significant and extensive changes. The current phase of change in health services offers all those working in maternity care an opportunity to develop these styles and practices. For such collaboration between midwives and doctors to develop successfully, several changes already underway need to continue, and deepen.

(a) Midwives should become the key professionals for women with low-risk pregnancies, a proposition now accepted by the Royal College of Obstetricians and Gynaecologists. Both their training and that of doctors should promote the communication skills necessary for new professional relationships (see below).

(b) All professionals must recognize that their involvement in maternity care may be different with different women, and in different pregnancies with the same woman.

(c) Women should be informed about the different roles that professionals might play during their pregnancy, to avoid them overvaluing the medical role. The fear that pregnancy is dangerous and can only be declared 'normal' in retrospect is a poorly informed medical perspective that is shared by many women (Raphael-Leff's 'regulators'), but it is exaggerated and needs alleviation. Journeys by car are also only safe in retrospect – they kill more women a year than pregnancy and childbirth – but do we seek medical guidance and surveillance whenever driving? The Dutch experience is that selection criteria developed in 1959 are adequate, with recent modification to incorporate new knowledge (Oppenheim 1993).

LESSONS FROM THE COMMUNITY

These three areas of change emphasize the primacy of good communication, flexible responses to people and situations, and a flow of information. Given the attitudes and practices that have developed, how can midwives and doctors now in post contribute to the development of a new approach to maternity care? In particular, what can those working in the community teach those working in hospital?

First, community staff may have less dysfunctional methods for overcoming anxiety than their hospital peers, and these methods might usefully be transferred. Group discussion and debriefing, if necessary by trained outsiders from clinical psychology or psychotherapy backgrounds, is an approach that has been used extensively in general practice training, and there are few young GPs who have not had some exposure to small group work, and to the methods and ideas of dynamic psychotherapy, in particular the Balint school. Paying attention to the emotional content of communication between people, as well as to the scientific basis of practice, and understanding how emotional communication facilitates or obstructs the work of professionals, have been the central themes of this style of education. Hospital specialists could learn much from it, given the high emotional charge in labour wards.

More active involvement of consultant staff in maternity units might do more than reduce the workload pressures on their juniors, but also create opportunities for support and education at an emotional level, if the consultants could acquire the same simple psychodynamic skills, as their GP peers. Specific training in communication skills, and in tolerance of uncertainty, has been developed in general practice using role-play techniques against a background culture that encourages reflection on consultation content. Inclusion of this approach in postgraduate training for obstetrics seems to us to be long overdue.

The close and continuing contact with the public that community staff experience cannot be replicated exactly in the hospital setting, but active user input to services is possible and desirable, both in provision of clinical support (especially for breast feeding, but in antenatal preparation too) and in policy-making. Opening the maternity units to the local groups of the National Childbirth Trust and the La Leche League may be a big step, but it would strengthen the relationships between units and the communities they seek to serve, and in a market environment this may even intensify 'brand loyalty'. The same user organizations may legitimately seek a voice at purchaser discussions about contracts with providers, and purchasing authorities could well augment their meagre sources of information about service quality through this route.

The debate about the safety of GP maternity units illustrates the antagonism that exists between hospital specialists and GPs. This has a long history (Honigsbaum 1979) and may be more unconscious than conscious until specific events bring it to the surface, but in our view it is a formidable obstacle to developing optimal care. The 'internal market' may well make these conflicts worse by promoting competition between maternity units themselves, and between general practice fundholders (who may soon find themselves managing the total budget for their population) with shrinking resources and expensive specialist services. Chapter 1 examines in more detail the issue of GP fundholders purchasing maternity care.

American experience of competition tends to encourage the loss of good, mission-driven, community-based care and the growth of better resourced but poorer quality, production-line services. Resisting this tendency by emphasizing the management element of the 'managed market' may be the most important contribution that those working in the community can make to the development of maternity services. Consistent input to the purchasing process, mobilization of both public and professional opinion around issues of quality of maternity care and systematic audit of local services are new and unfamiliar tasks that we must all undertake. Table 3.1 shows a first attempt at a purchaser's checklist for high-quality maternity care.

Table 3.1   A checklist for purchasing maternity care

- Patch-based community midwife teams with four to eight members provide 70% of antenatal care (with or without GP involvement), up to 80% of immediate postnatal care, a DOMINO facility and support for birth at home

- Antenatal care is dispersed as widely as possible in GPs' surgeries and health centres, along with specialist clinics for peripatetic obstetricians and parentcraft classes

- Voluntary organizations, especially the NCT, are involved in service provision where possible, and in policy-making

- Multidisciplinary workshops are a regular feature of continuing training of maternity service staff, under experienced external leadership

- Consultant expertise is available, both to hospital labour wards and to community services, at all times

- Adherence to published guidelines on obstetric practice

GP maternity units may continue to shrink in number, although their relatively low cost may appeal to purchasers and providers alike. We should not become preoccupied with the trend in GP maternity units, but instead focus on the contributions that GPs have made traditionally to antenatal care, and will begin to make to the planning and purchasing processes.

Birth at home may remain a fringe issue, supported by a few GPs with unusual relationships with local obstetricians and community midwives, and offered in some urban areas by the private sector, which will identify home birth as a fashionable niche market. The prospect for extension of the home birth option to a wider population probably depends on daring purchasers using their market powers to place contracts with so-called 'independent' midwives. Although this is happening in one area of South London, from what we have seen of purchasing authorities this seems unlikely to develop on a wide scale in the near future. However, it remains an outside possibility that could initiate the growth of an autonomous midwifery service comparable to that in The Netherlands, and similar to the National Maternity Service that predated the foundation of the NHS but failed to survive it (Peretz 1990). If such an organized form of autonomous midwifery emerged, would its practitioners work with GPs any more, or any better, than community midwives do now?

PRIMARY HEALTH CARE TEAMS

Teams and teamwork have been seen as the route to multiprofessional practice that brings together different skills for the benefit of the needy patient, client or customer. However, the idea of a 'primary health care team' including GP, midwife and health visitor, where different members play the key role in different circumstances, has been more talked about than practised. Primary health care teams (PHCTs) have not been successful for a variety of reasons: lack of knowledge about each other's roles; differences in training; different geographical organization; different management structures; and the prevailing political climate (Iliffe *et al.* 1993).

Perhaps the PHCT approach does not work in community obstetrics because there is no real need for it. Searching for the Holy Grail of multidisciplinary care structured in the form of a PHCT may be counterproductive, impossible or just plain unnecessary. A more realistic, science-based approach to interprofessional collaboration is needed to replace the ideologically driven commitment to PHCTs. Maternity care may be the area in which this realignment occurs first, if only because there is a critical mass of critical service users.

There is no ideal model for multidisciplinary maternity care. The teamwork needed for the inner-city area with high levels of deprivation in multilingual populations traumatized by past refugee experience and present experience of a racist society will not be the same as the 'independent' midwifery sought by an affluent and educated population for whom pregnancy is a 'stand alone' life event with designer symbolism. In the former the culturally attuned translator may be the key worker, displacing midwife and doctor, and in the latter the midwife may need only arms-length relationships with GPs in all but a few instances.

Between these extremes a variety of working relationships can develop, if we are all brave enough to allow them to. Perhaps the best approach to developing multidisciplinary maternity care would be to ask pregnant women what they want, before deciding on a professional agenda. A guess at a maternal agenda would be that most women would want information about the process of care, discussion of safety issues in the sense of knowing the real risks and the real benefits of suggested interventions, and a non-patronizing attitude amongst maternity staff. This would include simple prenatal counselling, simple early non-invasive anomaly diagnosis and more opportunity to discuss pregnancy and birth, along with less of the routine but unnecessary antenatal care, continuity of midwife care and unobtrusive but reliable medical support. Perhaps we should add having the baby in the way and in the place that suits the particular woman, on-going help with breast-feeding and the possibility of domestic support (Oppenheim 1993) to this list.

Of course, maternity care is more than the shallow ethos of consumerism, and professionals have a legitimate agenda. This agenda might include genetic counselling and screening, early anomaly diagnosis, focusing services on those women at risk, and a high level of collaboration and information transfer between professionals.

PROFESSIONAL EDUCATION

Can the decline of GP involvement in maternity care described by Smith and Jewell (1991) be averted? It is possible but would require a change in education for general practice obstetrics. At present most GPs gain their experience of obstetrics during a 6-month SHO post. During this time they are involved primarily in the management of abnormal pregnancies and labours. Many jobs are too busy for these SHOs to attend antenatal clinics in the community on a regular basis, where they could both learn about normal, uncomplicated pregnancy and appreciate the value of continuity of care. Most of their time will be spent on the labour ward dealing with distressed women or babies, where specific training in dealing with intense emotional distress takes second place – if it occurs at all – to the technical management of emergencies.

The inappropriateness of this training for those wanting to work in the community has been criticized from within medicine (Young 1991). Future GPs may not learn from their present obstetrics training why involvement in obstetric care will be both helpful to their patients and professionally rewarding. Opportunities to train doctors and midwives side by side need to be taken whenever they arise. Some involvement of junior doctors in the management of abnormal pregnancy and labour is vital if they are going to be a useful support in the community, but they also need to learn the normal process and outcome of labour.

One way of overcoming this unbalanced experience would be to attach junior doctors to midwives for part of their training on the labour ward, rather than to the obstetric registrar. They would then become familiar with birth as a normal process sometimes needing intervention but always needing support, rather than a process that was decreed 'normal' only in retrospect. GPs involved in maternity care soon learn that their presence during pregnancy and labour can confirm normality, provide support for the relatives, increase continuity and confidence and provide a response to developing risks. There is no reason why this cannot be learned in the hospital context, in our view. Only when doctors put normal pregnancy and birth at the centre of their thinking will they be able to find an appropriate place in community-based maternity care.

Early reports on GP obstetrics did not recognize the differences between training needs for GPs and career obstetricians (RCOG/RCGP 1982) although later recommendations have tried to address this area (RCOG/RCGP 1991). Changing the teaching and organization of hospital obstetrics to accommodate new training styles would be expensive in the first instance, because more doctors would be needed in junior obstetric jobs and more specialists would have to roll their sleeves up, but if the outcome is an obstetric workforce that is more patient-centred and more emotionally experienced then such an investment may well be cost effective in the longer term.

The Diploma of the Royal College of Obstetricians and Gynaecologists is the examination designed to test the obstetric skills of GPs. Whilst it remains hospital-oriented, it should be reconfigured to make it more appropriate to general practice obstetrics and its acquisition should be a precondition for a GP role in community obstetrics. Because obstetric knowledge changes, re-accreditation of GP obstetricians is essential. At the very least, attendance at a refresher course on obstetrics every 5 years should become mandatory for all GP obstetricians, but with a curriculum appropriate to the task, and perhaps in a multiprofessional setting. Arguably, annual reports from general practice should include audits of pregnancy outcomes for the practice population, and descriptions of the level of GP involvement.

The present payment system for GPs involved in maternity care is unnecessarily complex, reflects a role that is incompatible with a midwife led service, and encourages GPs to undertake unnecessary work simply because they are paid for it, whilst leaving midwives to get on with the real hard graft. For example, GPs are paid for up to five postnatal visits for each woman, and some do them, even though this effort duplicates the visits of the community midwife and potentially increases the amount of contradictory and confusing information received by the new mother.

Whilst postnatal visits may improve the relationship between the woman and her doctor, this is the excuse for doing them, not the true reason. Frequent visiting of the ill and disabled is uncommon, although probably more important to the ill and disabled than are postnatal visits, but it is not lucrative. A sensible payment system for GP obstetrics would be a form of bonus paid to the practice for running maternity services, with audits of the process of antenatal and postnatal care being produced as evidence of activity. Provision of intra-partum care, special approaches to particularly vulnerable groups, or extra resources committed to, say, promotion of breast feeding could attract a higher level of bonus.

CONCLUSIONS

An opportunity exists for the development of multidisciplinary maternity care in the community. Opportunities for innovative practice may increase as the NHS apparatus with its efforts at a standardized service dissolves into locally controlled units that seek public recognition. On the other hand, the purchaser–provider split with Trusts and fundholder units jostling for business could also make maternity care more problematic for women, because the market has the habit of letting large, potent corporate organizations with a pro-duction-line approach to clinical practice drive small, locality-based and mission-driven services out of business.

In a worst-case scenario the public sector maternity services will dwindle to hard-pressed and under-resourced labour wards with community outreach teams, just able to process pregnant women with low incomes. The better off will opt for 'independent' (private) midwives working from, or at least along-side, private hospitals where there will be at least the outward display of a woman-centred approach to natural 'birthing', or perhaps with GP fundholders as an income-generating arm of the practice. In the more optimistic perspective that we have tried to outline, community-based maternity care will increase its influence over hospital maternity units, and careful collaboration between pro-fessionals, and between hospital and community services, will alter the culture of maternity care at local level.

Many people have an interest in change and development in maternity care, and we have grounds for optimism despite the current destabilization of the NHS. We believe that the small efforts made by many doctors, midwives and articulate, involved women will have a cumulative effect on the quality of maternity care, and act as a brake on the destructive tendencies of the medical market. Some efforts seem particularly important. Changes are needed in medi-cal education, especially at the postgraduate level, to refocus medical experience and emotion on normality. Accreditation and payment of GP obstetricians needs to change, to enhance clinical skills and abolish perverse financial incentives.

Communication of what is meant by 'continuity of care', and why it matters for pregnancy, birth and parenting, seems necessary, if only as an antidote to superficial and infantile ideas about consumerism. Experimentation in organiz-ation and user involvement needs promotion, and different experiences need to be publicized and constructively discussed. The search for one model of organ-ization for community maternity services can be abandoned in favour of prag-matic solutions that allow pregnant women to write the first draft of the maternity agenda. Finally, and above all, the interest and pressure groups, derided by the medical establishment as 'trendy' and 'middle class', which have done so much to change maternity services (in balance, for the better), deserve professional support and encouragement.

REFERENCES

Balla, J.I., Elstein, A.S. and Christensen, C. (1989) Obstacles to acceptance of clinical decision analysis, *British Medical Journal* **298:** 579.

Barrett, J.F.R., Jarvis, G.J., Macdonald, H.N., Buchan, P.C., Tyrell, S.N. and Lilford, R.J. (1990) Inconsistencies in clinical decisions in obstetrics, *Lancet* **336:** 549.

Bryce, F.C., Clayton, J.K., Rand, R.J., Beck, I., Farquarson, D.I.M. and Jones, S.E. (1990) General practitioner obstetrics in Bradford, *British Medical Journal* **300:** 725.

Bull, M.J.V. (1988) General practice obstetrics . . . is there a future? *Update* **37:** 590.

Campbell, R. and Macfarlane, A. (1987) *Where to be Born; the Debate and the Evidence*, Oxford: National Perinatal Epidemiology Unit.

Cardozo, L. (1993) Is routine induction of labour at term ever justified? *British Medical Journal* **306:** 840.

Cumberlege, J. (1993) *Changing Childbirth, Report of the Expert Maternity Group*, London: HMSO.

Dawes, M.G., Green, J. and Ashurst, H. (1992) Routine weighing in pregnancy, *British Medical Journal* **304:** 487.

Flint, C., Pailengeris, P. and Grant, A. (1989) The 'know your midwife' scheme – a randomised trial of continuity of care by a team of midwives, *Midwifery* **5:** 11.

Ford, C., Iliffe, S. and Franklin, O. (1991) Outcome of planned home births in an inner city practice, *British Medical Journal* **302:** 1517.

Hall, M. (1993) Rituals in antenatal care – do we need them? *British Medical Journal* **307:** 697.

Hall, M.K., Chung, P.K. and MacGillivray, I. (1980) Is routine antenatal care worthwhile? *Lancet* **1:** 78.

Honigsbaum, F. (1979) *The Division in British Medicine: a History of the Separation of General Practice from Hospital Care 1911–1968*, London: Kogan Page.

Huntingford, P. (1980) Obstetrics – whose baby? *Medicine in Society* **6(1):** 24.

Iliffe, S., Gilbert, A., Pearson, P. *et al.* (1993) *Teams and Teamwork*, London: Medical World/Health Visitor.

Jewell, D. and Smith, L. (1990) Is there a future for general practitioner obstetrics? In *RCGP Members Reference Book*, p. 239, London: RCGP.

Johnson, D.B. (1990) General practice obstetrics in Bradford, *British Medical Journal* **300:** 874.

Kitzinger, S. (1988) *The Midwife Challenge*, London: Pandora Press.

Klein, M., Lloyd, I., Redman, C. *et al.* (1993) A comparison of low risk pregnant women booked for delivery in two systems of care: shared care (consultant) and integrated practice unit, *British Journal of Obstetrics and Gynaecology* **90:** 118.

Loudon, I. (1990) Obstetrics and the general practitioner, *British Medical Journal* **301:** 705.

Marsh, G.N. (1982) The speciality of general practice obstetrics, *Lancet* **1:** 669.

Marsh, G.N. (1985) General practice participation in the Northern Region in 1983, *British Medical Journal* **290:** 973.

Marsh, G.N. (1991) Antenatal care for the 1990s, In *RCGP Members Reference Book*, p. 429, London: RCGP.

Nielson, J.P. (1993) Cardiotocography during labour, *British Medical Journal* **306:** 347.

Oakley, A. (1979) *From Here to Maternity*, London: Pelican Books.

Oppenheim, C. (1993) Organising midwifery led care in The Netherlands, *British Medical Journal* **307:** 1400.

Peretz, E. (1990) A maternity service for England and Wales. In Garcia, J., Kilpatrick, R. and Richards, M. (eds) *The Politics of Maternity Care*, p. 30, Oxford: Clarendon.

Raphael-Leff, J. (1991) *Psychological Processes of Child-bearing*, London: Chapman & Hall.

RCOG/RCGP (1982) Joint working party of the Royal College of Obstetrics and Royal College of General Practitioners: report on training for obstetrics and gynaecology for general practitioners, *Journal of the Royal College of General Practice* **32:** 116.

RCOG/RCGP (1991) Report on training for obstetrics and gynaecology for general practitioners. *Journal of the Royal College of General Practice* **32:** 116.

Sangala, V., Dunster, G., Bohin, S. and Osborne, J.P. (1990) Perinatal mortality rates in isolated general practitioner units, *British Medical Journal* **301:** 418.

Smith, L.F.P. (1990) Quality, continuity and maternity care, In *RCGP Members Reference Book*, p. 239, London: RCGP.

Smith, L.F.P. and Jewell, D. (1991) Contribution of general practitioners to hospital intra-partum care in maternity units in England and Wales in 1988, *British Medical Journal* **302:** 13.

Street, P., Gannon, M.J. and Holt, E.M. (1991) Community obstetrics care in West Berkshire, *British Medical Journal* **302:** 698.

Tew, M. (1985) Place of birth and perinatal mortality, *Journal of the Royal College of General Practitioners* **35:** 390.

Treffers, P.E., Eskes, M., Kleiverda, G. *et al.* (1990) Home births and minimal medical interventions, *Journal of the American Medical Association* **204:** 2206.

Van Alten, D., Eskes, M. and Treffers, P.E. (1989) Midwifery in The Netherlands. The Wormeveer study: selection, mode of delivery, perinatal mortality and infant morbidity, *British Journal of Obstetrics & Gynaecology* **96:** 656.

Waterston, T. and Davies, J. (1993) Could hospitals do more to encourage breast feeding? *British Medical Journal* **307:** 1437.

Winterton, N. (1992) *House of Commons Health Committee Report on Maternity Services*, London: HMSO.

Young, G. (1991) General practice and the future of obstetric care, *British Journal of General Practice* **41**: 266.

Zander, L. and Chamberlain, G. (1984) *Pregnancy Care for the 1980s*, London: Royal Society of Medicine.

4

The Potential of Postnatal Care

Jo Garcia and Sally Marchant

INTRODUCTION

This chapter looks at the statutory and clinical background to postnatal home visiting by midwives, and then describes the range of current visiting policies in England and Wales using information from research carried out by the National Perinatal Epidemiology Unit (NPEU) over the last 4 years. This research has provided information about policies and practices in postnatal care, looking mainly at the structure and organization of care rather than at detailed clinical care. Other research on postnatal health and health care is described in order to explore the purpose of postnatal home visiting in current midwifery care. The chapter concludes with some suggestions for evaluation and audit in postnatal care.

STATUTE AND REGULATION

The current regulation of the midwife's practice in the postnatal period is through statute in the Midwife's Rules (UKCC 1991). In conjunction with these, there is the Midwife's Code of Practice, which is a set of non-statutory guidelines to good midwifery practice. The World Health Organization (WHO) definition and activities of a midwife in the Midwife's Code of Practice set out the role of the midwife in the postnatal period as carer and adviser to the newly delivered mother and baby. The practices of the midwife may also extend into gynaecological and family planning aspects of care (UKCC 1994).

A review of the Handbooks and Codes written for midwives after the passing of the Midwives Act in 1902 up to the current edition illustrates how the role of the midwife and the instructions for midwifery care in the postnatal period have changed. A 1919 edition of the *Handbook for Midwives*, which incorporated the Rules of the Central Midwives' Board (1919), identifies duties to the mother in the lying-in period, which was defined as:

in a normal case to mean the time occupied from the labour and a period of 10 days thereafter.

The midwife shall be responsible for:

the cleanliness, and shall give all necessary directions for securing the comfort and proper dieting of the mother and child during the lying-in period.

In addition the midwife was required to send for medical help in cases of abnormality or complication. For the lying-in period these were listed as:

- fits or convulsions;
- abdominal swelling or tenderness;
- offensive lochia, if persistent;
- rigor with raised temperature;
- rise of temperature above 100.4°F with quickening of the pulse for more than 24 h;
- unusual swelling of the breasts with local tenderness or pain;
- secondary postpartum haemorrhage;
- white leg.

Following the 1902 Midwives Act, the profession of midwifery was recognized by statute, and midwifery training approved. For several years following this there were certified midwives and untrained 'handywomen' who still gave midwifery care, especially in the country districts. Although, in the 1919 Handbook, the midwife is given responsibility for ensuring reasonable conditions of cleanliness and nutrition for the mother, certified midwives were unlikely to actually clean or cook as the untrained midwives had done previously.

Prior to 1918, in situations where the midwife needed to call for medical aid, it was often left to the midwife to settle the doctor's fee if the family were unable to pay. Following the 1918 Act this became the responsibility of the local supervising authorities. The list of symptoms that necessitated referral are largely concentrated around those of infection and circulatory problems, the main causes of maternal mortality at the time (Donnison 1988).

By 1935 (Central Midwives' Board 1935) the duties of the midwife to the patient (sic) had been added to and made more specific. In addition to the general supervision during the lying-in period mentioned in 1919, the midwife was now told that:

If a rise in temperature (or any other condition requiring close supervision) be found at the morning visit, an evening visit must be paid, unless the midwife is relieved from the obligation by the Local Supervising Authority.

This suggests that normal domiciliary practice was to visit daily, rather than to be in more constant attendance. There is also more detailed attention to record-keeping and procedures to counter infection. The list of complications had also been elaborated, perhaps reflecting increased concern about maternal morbidity. Changes were made to the definition of raised temperature so that a 'rise of temperature to 100.4°F for 24 hours or its recurrence within that period, or a rise in temperature above 99.4°F on three successive days' should now lead to a call for medical aid. In addition a 'steadily rising pulse rate' was also listed and secondary postpartum haemorrhage was replaced by 'excessive or prolonged bleeding'.

The 1952 Handbook (Central Midwives' Board 1952) includes several definitions of key terms in midwifery. The lying-in period was now:

a period being not less than 14 days nor more than 28 days after the end of the labour during which the continued attendance of the midwife on the mother and child is requisite.

This is noteworthy firstly because of its clear statement of the midwife's responsibility and also because, apart from the reduction from 14 to 10 postnatal days, this definition has remained substantially unchanged to the present day. By this date the midwife's duties in the postnatal period were set out very clearly:

. . . it is expected that the midwife will normally pay morning and evening visits for the first few days after delivery, but if a rise of temperature (or any other condition requiring close supervision) be found at the morning visit, an evening visit must be paid unless the midwife is relieved from the obligation by the local supervising author-ity. The midwife must take the pulse rate and temperature of the patient at each visit and must enter her records accurately, with dates and times, in the form of a pulse and temperature chart approved by the Board, such form being carefully preserved.

Instead of the list of abnormalities requiring referral to a doctor, as given in earlier years, any case of illness in the mother or child is said to require referral. However, specific instructions about raised temperature remain in the text for the postnatal period.

There was little change in these sections of the handbooks for the next 25 years, apart from a clearer separation of the Midwives' Rules and the Midwife's Code of Practice. An extract from the Code of Practice for 1978 states (Central Midwives' Board 1978):

The midwife shall be responsible for the welfare of the mother and baby during the postnatal period. In domiciliary practice it is expected that the midwife will normally pay morning and evening visits for the first few days after delivery, but if any condition requiring close supervision be found at the morning visit, an evening visit must be paid unless the midwife is relieved from the obligation by the appropriate authority. The midwife must take the pulse rate and temperature of the patient at each visit and make the detailed observations necessary to assess maternal progress. She must record her findings and observations on each visit, entering the date, time and signature in the patient's records.

The Nurses, Midwives and Health Visitors Act of 1979 led to the setting up of the United Kingdom Central Council for Nurses, Midwives and Health Visitors (UKCC) as a statutory body to regulate the professions. This was composed of elected and appointed members drawn more representatively from the profession. Revision of the Midwife's Rules and the Midwife's Code of Practice by the Midwifery committee of the UKCC has continued on a regular basis. After 1986 the Code of Practice (UKCC 1986) became less precise, especially in clinical instruction such as the timing, number and content of postnatal visits. The directive about daily visiting was removed and guidance about referral to a doctor in the case of abnormality also became more general. In the current edition of the Midwife's Rules the postnatal period is defined as:

a period of not less than ten and not more than twenty-eight days after the end of labour, during which the continued attendance of a midwife upon the mother and baby is requisite.

(UKCC 1993)

Removal of the more detailed instructions for care previously given in the Code of Practice appeared to give rise to some confusion between the statutory responsibilities of the midwife and the regulation of the midwife's practice, for example the pattern for visits in the postnatal period. This resulted in the United Kingdom Central Council for Nursing, Midwifery and Health Visiting clarifying the definition of the postnatal period given in the Midwives' Rules in a letter to the profession (UKCC 1992):

each midwife is personally responsible and accountable for the exercise of professional judgement and determining appropriate practice in relation to mother and baby. This, naturally, includes judgements about the number of visits and any additional visits required in the postnatal period.

The extracts from the handbook and rules over the last 70 years illustrate that whereas statute has changed very little, the Code of Practice has changed considerably in focus and content. There may also be an element of increased freedom for the individual midwife who no longer has the constraints of the specified duties, but responsibility for midwifery care in an appropriate setting. The impact of the most recent changes in the Code of Practice is covered next.

CURRENT POLICIES ON UK POSTNATAL HOME VISITING

At the end of the 1980s it appeared that there was a change from a policy of routine daily visiting up to the 10th postnatal day, to policies that allowed midwives to miss one or two visits before the 10th day if appropriate. There was no good information, though, about the extent to which these new policies were coming into force.

This led to a survey of English health districts which was carried out in 1991 and which focused on two main topics: policies about the organization of antenatal care for different categories of women, and policies and practices concerning postnatal home visiting by community midwives. It is these latter data that will be referred to in this chapter. The whole survey is described in more detail elsewhere (Garcia *et al.* 1994).

The survey showed that by 1991, almost all districts had a policy of selective visits to mothers at home before the 10th postnatal day. In only 10 districts was the traditional policy of daily visiting still being followed. In 10 further districts this policy was still followed but was under review, or change was under discussion, and in another nine the practice had changed even though the formal policy had not. Most districts (137, 81%) had changed their policy to one of selective visiting. In addition, policies in almost all districts (158/170) specified that midwives should visit after the 10th day as they judged necessary, with a few (10) reporting visits on specific days after the 10th day, and only two indicating that visiting after the 10th day was unusual.

Although almost all those who responded to our questionnaire indicated that they had adopted selective visiting, some of the policies that were described gave far more scope to the midwife's judgement than others. In some places the policy gave the midwife the power to plan an agreed pattern of visits with the mother, while in others, visits could be missed on only one or two specified days. In general we found very little discussion about what it meant to visit selectively and what criteria might be used to judge who should be visited. This raises questions about the content and organization of postnatal care.

WHAT ARE THE PURPOSES OF POSTNATAL CARE?

Safeguarding maternal health

Over the last few years, the postnatal period has begun to receive more attention from policy makers, researchers, care-givers and voluntary groups. There is now more information from research about postnatal health and health care (Glazener *et al.* 1993). One finding from recent research is that women are often left with problems in the postnatal period that may be long lasting. A study of the health of women following childbirth identified that 47% of women developed at least one health problem lasting more than 6 weeks within the first 3 months after delivery of the baby (MacArthur *et al.* 1991). This is supported by evidence from a study on postnatal care in one region in Scotland, which showed that 87% of postnatal women had at least one health problem once they were at home, 46% of these being major problems of bleeding or high blood pressure, and 78% relatively minor problems such as tiredness, backache, constipation, piles or headache (Glazener *et al.* 1993).

Postnatal care has the potential to alleviate some of the burden of physical and psychological ill health for mothers (Glazener *et al.* 1993). There is evidence, for example, that appropriate help at the right time can help to prevent or reduce postnatal depression (Holden *et al.* 1989, Holden 1990). In addition, because all but a tiny number of postnatal women in the UK are visited by a midwife (Murphy-Black 1989), postnatal care provides an important opportunity for women's concerns about their health to be addressed.

The postnatal period is a complex time which involves the mother in sometimes major changes, psychological as well as physical. The midwife has a responsibility to oversee the health of the mother and baby and to give support and advice. The care set out in one current textbook widely used for the education of student midwives (Bennett and Brown 1993) illustrates the dependence of this aspect of midwifery care on traditional and routine practices. A chapter is devoted to the physiology, psychology and management of the puerperium. This chapter gives detailed information on the physiology of the structures likely to be affected following childbirth. The 'management' part of the chapter looks at the health of the mother and her recovery following childbirth and describes the format of a physical examination. This lists what is to be observed or tested as part of the check in quite a formalized way, noting normal or possible abnormal findings.

Midwives may use midwifery records which set out every system identified in the postnatal check in the form of a table or list, and just a short response in the form of a tick or single word is required to verify that the check has been completed. A procedure that works through a set pattern in this way aims to identify the return to normal or otherwise of systems or structures affected in pregnancy and labour. Currently this approach is used indiscriminately for all women. This means that in the absence of a clear need for referral to a medical practitioner, it is the midwife who decides whether a woman needs more attention, such as spending longer with mothers who have had traumatic deliveries or have social problems, as well as identifying those who may need less support.

This routine work of midwives in the postnatal period is, however, largely based on the detection of disease or of screening for pathological problems such as secondary postpartum haemorrhage or virulent infection. Although these are still major causes of maternal morbidity in the developing world they would appear to have less importance for most mothers in the developed world where secondary postpartum haemorrhage, for example, occurs in less than 1% of the population (ACOG Technical Bulletin 1990). Before the introduction of antibiotics earlier this century, the presence of uterine sepsis accounted for a very high proportion of maternal deaths (Loudon 1986) and this is possibly why such importance is still placed on the daily postnatal examination.

The current principal causes of maternal death in the UK are thrombosis and thromboembolism, hypertensive disorders of pregnancy and haemorrhage (Report of the Confidential Enquiry into Maternal Deaths in the United Kingdom 1988–90). Some of these conditions can be identified before the postnatal period. The mother's general state of health and the pre-existing evidence of disease or disorder may alert care-givers to women at risk, rather than working on the basis that the whole population of postnatal women is at risk.

There are other forms of morbidity that interfere with the process of adaptation to motherhood and could increase the likelihood of feelings of low esteem or depression postnatally. A high proportion of breastfeeding mothers suffer morbidity from poor positioning at the breast and resultant sore nipples, and infection in the breast (White *et al.* 1992). Perineal trauma resulting from episiotomies, tears or bruising may affect the mother's ability to sit or walk comfortably and poorly healed perineal tissue may affect the sexual relations between a couple for months after the birth (Sleep 1991).

The needs of the postnatal mother in the UK have changed from those of 70 years ago, and the care provided and observations made by midwives should reflect this. Re-evaluation of the purpose of postnatal visiting might look more towards reducing the occurrence of morbidity, which affects the ability of the mother to return to reasonable health, rather than screening everyone for serious outcomes, which affect only a few. This will include identifying pre-existing factors for those at high risk of serious disease, referral to other agencies when necessary and making provision for psychological and social support where this is needed.

Providing social and personal support for women and families

There is a traditional view that despite education in the antenatal period for post-natal events, many parents feel ill-equipped to care for the newly born infant. The role of the midwife in the first postnatal days has shifted more towards meeting these needs with a view to increasing the parents' own confidence in their abilities to cope when they need to, on their own. The midwife has an important role to play in supporting women who choose to breastfeed and have not had experience of breastfeeding before. The midwife has a responsibility to see that social conditions are suitable for both the mother and the new baby and this may involve liaison with social services. Health education information is appropriate at this time both to help to avoid ill health in the baby and to raise mothers' awareness about their health and health care. There is evidence that many women do not seek professional help for problems in the postnatal period (MacArthur *et al.* 1991) so common physical and psychological problems can be raised by the midwife and issues such as the need for cervical smears and the use of adequate contraception discussed. Although some of these areas may be covered by giving out leaflets and booklets, the work of the midwife visiting the mother at home involves practical demonstrations of infant care and being present while the parents seek reassurance about their own competence.

In looking at the attention women need at this time it is possible to assume that it falls almost entirely to the midwife to assess the mother's health, to provide education and to give advice for child care. Although the midwife is the primary care-giver in the early stages, she is supported by the general practitioner (GP) and later transfers care to the health visitor. The lines of responsibility between care-givers in the postnatal period can become confused as the midwife may visit for up to 28 days after the birth (Robinson *et al.* 1983). In the absence of any complications it is usual for the health visitor to assume care for the mother shortly after the 10th postnatal day and for women to be followed-up through community or GP clinics. In the past, screening for physical problems was central to the purpose of the midwife's visit and provided a clear identity for the role of the midwife in the postnatal period in both the hospital and the mother's own home. With increasing awareness of the need for psychological and social support and parent and health education, the relative roles of midwife and health visitor could become blurred.

The benefits of social and psychological support have been supported by research in specific aspects of maternity care such as care in labour (Hodnett 1994) and postnatal depression (Holden 1990). Midwives (and health visitors) need to look at these aspects of their work in the light of the evidence, and map out what they hope to achieve with the support they offer. Research may be needed to demonstrate the value of other aspects of their care (health promotion, general support, contact with parent networks, etc.) and the best ways of providing care that has been shown to be effective.

Caring for the whole person

Midwives do have the opportunity to provide care that meets the physical and psychological needs of women and families. In addition, midwifery care in the community reaches all types of families, including those who clearly have extra needs and those who do not appear to need help, but may have needs that are not recognized. The problem is that all aspects of health care are under scrutiny, and community midwifery care is relatively expensive. We do not have much information about what midwives do in the course of a postnatal home visit, nor do we know much about which aspects of care are likely to be useful to mothers. Midwifery postnatal care needs to have clear objectives and be supported by good evidence about the components of care and the organization of provision.

QUESTIONS ABOUT THE CURRENT ORGANIZ-ATION OF MIDWIFERY CARE IN THE COMMUNITY

The balance between antenatal, intrapartum and postnatal work

It is only comparatively recently that attention has been paid to the organization and content of the postnatal visit and the work of the midwife in the community. This is possibly because of a general reorganization of care schemes such as the introduction of team midwifery, and increased demands on health-care providers to undertake audit of both clinical outcomes and the use of resources. Postnatal visiting in the home is time-consuming and expensive in terms of professional expertise and health service resources. Shorter stays in hospital can increase the work of community visiting in the postnatal period. In many places midwives working in the community are taking on new tasks such as home bookings and may be eager to carry out more intrapartum care, both at home and in hospital. They may experience some conflict between the various aspects of their role in dealing with priorities of acute situations such as being with a woman in labour with those of helping women breastfeed.

Community midwives interviewed as part of the NPEU Postnatal Care Project illustrate some of the changes taking place in postnatal home visiting. The NPEU Postnatal Care Project was a descriptive study started in 1990 (Garcia and Marchant 1992). It concentrated on one English Health Region and described the services offered to women in the postnatal period in all the districts in that region. There followed an in-depth study of the care and postnatal health of nearly 200 women who were recruited from two of those districts. This study gives a view of the services provided from the viewpoint of the caregivers, and quite detailed information from the women about their health and the care they received following the delivery and up to 8 weeks postnatally.

Midwives from the 16 districts covered in the first part of the study were interviewed about the organization of postnatal care. The midwives spoke of an increased workload through shorter postnatal hospital stays for mothers and an expansion of their role in the community, which appeared to affect the number and content of the visits.

We try to visit all women antenatally – all are our clients regardless of whether they are domino or not, and postnatal care is better if we know them.

Bits are added on all the time. We are seeing [women who have had] *miscarriages now.*

[Postnatal] visits need more haemoglobin bloods, etc., taking longer and (there is) more antenatal care.

The pattern of care postnatally

Once the newly delivered mother is at home, the midwife in the community is responsible for the whole range of care for the mother and baby, and is traditionally required to fit this in with the standard format of visits. Some Districts have maintained daily visiting to the 10th day and others have changed, or were in the process of changing, to visiting on a more flexible basis. One reason given for changing to selective visiting is to reduce the number of midwives that a woman sees postnatally. A midwife said:

You do the first one (visit) then decide. You try to give continuity – that's new in the last six months. Now we couldn't *do (visit) everyone to the 10th day.*

If all is well we discharge them on the 9th–10th day. If not we go on as we decide. For about half the women, I go in after the 10th day. Its hard to stop when they know me.

Midwives may need to prioritize the components of the midwifery care required for each visit, which will now include more teaching of the care of a newborn baby and more supervision with feeding in the early days. The care of low-birth-weight babies and babies who develop jaundice once they are at home may require more specialized skills and be a departure from a more task-orientated form of routine care.

Outside the UK, it is unusual for the midwife to make routine unsolicited home visits over a period as long as 10 days. In some parts of Europe, a midwife will visit for a few days and then be available for contact by the mother in the first 10–14 days (personal communication, G. Jaskowsky). In America and Canada routine care is offered in hospital with just one or two visits in the home, sometimes several days after discharge. Various studies that have looked at the effect of the trend to shorter stays in hospital in the postnatal period have identified that mothers were missing out on the care, especially the teaching of parent skills, that they would normally receive. Many of the North American early discharge programmes are intended to be supplementary to hospital post-natal care, and emphasize education for parenthood rather than the physical recovery from the effects of pregnancy and birth (Norr and Nacion 1987).

The home visiting patterns that are currently routine in the UK could be viewed as a practice that has survived from the old lying-in period and which continues by default rather than design. There is a considerable difference in the position of women within society now in comparison with the earlier part of this century. Women were then more likely to have witnessed child care and early infancy, particularly breast feeding, within the family around them. There is less opportunity for this now, because families are smaller and breastfeeding is a more private affair. When women return to work a few months after the birth, there is less opportunity to learn from other mothers. Changes in the family network also lead to women not being able to rely on the support of their own mothers or other female family members because they may live some distance away or may be in full-time work. This can lead to women feeling isolated in the postnatal period, with limited access to support networks.

For women who have deliveries in hospital, the length of stay is now more likely to suit the needs and choice of the mothers, in preference to those of the institution. However, this is not always the case and where bed space for post-natal women is limited, those women who may need extra time in hospital for other than medical reasons may find this unavailable.

Routine or selective care?

Nursing and midwifery have tended to include a substantial amount of routine practice, often coupled with the allocation of care-givers to tasks rather than to individuals (Walsh and Ford 1989). Routines may be vital to the safe organiz-ation of care for groups of people, especially when those receiving care are ill and less able to identify and ask for what they need. However, routine care can be wasteful and inflexible, and may increase the chance of iatrogenic problems when tests or interventions are applied unnecessarily (Garforth and Garcia 1989). Individual components of care can no longer be accepted without question, and this is true for the more 'minor' tests and treatments as well as the important new techniques. Nursing researchers are looking in detail at basic aspects of their care such as temperature measurement (Clayton 1987), and similar questions are being asked in midwifery (Garforth and Garcia 1989, Garcia and Marchant 1992, Montgomery and Alexander 1994).

The introduction of more individualized care – the nursing or midwifery process – was intended to improve the relevance of care to the individual, and to make care more personal, more efficient and more satisfying for staff. Individualized care does not in itself conflict with regular monitoring or treatment routines, but should allow the care-giver to exercise greater judgement within agreed policies and respond to the person who is being cared for.

There is a statutory requirement in the Midwives' Rules for midwives to document fully the care that they give. Prescribed forms may provide evidence about the health of an individual related to routine observations taken contemporaneously. However, it is rare for any discussion or advice given about either the mother's or the baby's health, care or feeding to be written down for the mother to refer to at a later time. Midwifery records may therefore be seen as representing the interests of the midwife rather than informing the mother about the content of the visit or state of her health.

What are the potential advantages and disadvantages of selective postnatal home visiting? Selective visiting could allow midwives to concentrate their efforts where they are most needed, releasing more time for those women who have particular problems. It has the potential to improve continuity of carer, because the midwife that a woman knows need not be replaced by another just to achieve a visit every day for 10 days. This may be particularly important in view of the common complaints about conflicting advice in the postnatal period (Garcia 1989, Green *et al.* 1988).

Continuing a pattern of daily visiting, on the other hand, may bring the midwife into contact with women who are not good at saying what they need and who might be reluctant to ask for a visit or phone for advice. Access to a telephone is important if women are to be able to take advantage of midwifery support in the community, without midwifery visits taking place on a routine basis. There may be clinical reasons why care should be provided on certain days, for example in order to carry out tests on the mother or baby at the most appropriate time, or for those mothers with increased risks of postnatal complications.

Midwifery care needs to respond to the individual circumstances of the postnatal mother, rather than rely on routine which is imposed on women and midwives. For example, some women will need greater levels of support because of their social background, whereas others may need medical support in the form of continued analgesia for pain. To achieve a responsive form of care requires a flexibility that should be at its best when midwives are visiting postnatal women at home. The time taken for a visit and the components of that visit should be influenced by the particular circumstances of the mother, baby and family. Rigid adherence to similarly rigid policies would not seem to serve the purposes of the midwife as educator and advisor.

RESEARCH AND AUDIT IN POSTNATAL CARE

One approach to the assessment of maternity care is to look at the individual tests and treatments that make up the care and ask whether each is justified, when, and for which women. This has begun to be done for antenatal care by looking at the normal schedule of care and asking about the possible benefits of that timetable, and of the individual tests such as blood pressure measurement or ultrasound (Hall *et al.* 1985). For the postnatal period, though, there is little work that describes the content of care; the effectiveness and appropriate use of the components of care are still more neglected. Ultimately the aim of research will be to build up an appropriate pattern of care in a rational way on the basis of effective tests and treatments. In the absence of much of this groundwork we can still look critically at the pattern of care, and attempt to answer some of the questions raised in the preceding paragraph.

A recent 'before and after' study of home visiting in Glasgow (Twaddle *et al.* 1993) showed that a change from routine daily visiting to a more flexible, individualized form of care led to an improvement in continuity of carer. Women were just as satisfied with the new form of care. Although few places will now be considering whether to change from routine to selective visiting, it is clear from the findings of our survey of local policies that the term 'selective visiting' covers a wide range of patterns of care. There is certainly scope for different approaches to postnatal home visiting to be explored in research and audit.

As a minimum it is useful to describe the care that is being given. For example, the NPEU Postnatal Care Project can compare the pattern of postnatal care that the mothers received in the two districts. Figures 4.1 and 4.2 show, for the two districts, the proportions of women in hospital, at home and visited by a midwife, and at home without a visit from a midwife, for each of the first 14 days after the birth. The districts differed in their policies on length of hospital stay and on selective visiting before the 10th day. In district 1, lengths of stay were still expected to be fairly long, and a policy of daily visiting to the 10th day was still in place. In district 2, lengths of stay had been reduced and there was a selective policy for home visiting. These charts show the some-

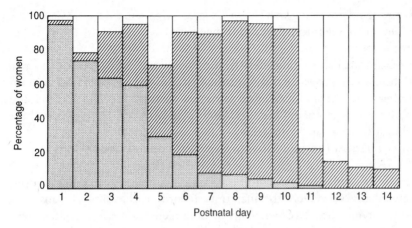

Figure 4.1 Visiting patterns for District 1: ▥, hospital; ▨, home, visited; ▢, home, not visited. Excludes 11 women for whom full visiting pattern was not known (n=121).

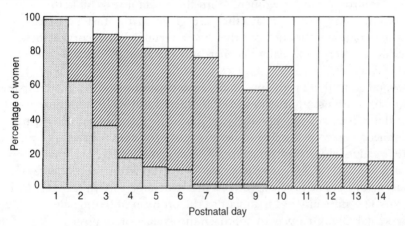

Figure 4.2 Visiting patterns for District 2: ▥, hospital; ▨, home, visited; ▢, home, not visited. Excludes 8 women for whom full visiting pattern was not known (n=58).

what shorter lengths of stay in district 2, although the contrast is not as marked as the approach in the two places might suggest. From the viewpoint of the work for a midwife in the community, more women in district 2 are at home on days 3 and 4, and most of them are being visited. Women in district 2 are less likely to be visited at home on days 7–10, but somewhat more likely to have a visit after day 10. Other results from this survey, which is being analysed at the moment, will be able to throw more light on the pattern of visiting in the two districts, from the viewpoint of midwives and mothers.

In addition to describing the pattern of postnatal care, two other audit questions can be asked:

- Are standards being met?
- Does care seem to be related to need?

First, are standards being met? If, for example, a policy states that the midwife should visit twice each day for the first 3 days, or should continue to visit a mother until the umbilical cord separates, then we can check to see if these are followed in practice. Of course some standards will have to have been set for this question to make sense.

Does care seem to be related to need? We can ask which sorts of mothers are visited more often or for longer. Are they those likely to need extra help, or are they perhaps those who are 'easier' to visit. This could be done by reviewing retrospectively the maternity records at the time of transfer home and identifying those women who meet agreed criteria as being at increased risk of postnatal problems, perhaps because of the type of delivery or social needs. The subsequent care given to these women could then be compared with a 'control' group of women. With these data it is possible to do analyses of this kind, and also to relate the care given in the first postnatal days to women's comments about how they were feeling. We recorded these comments using a very short daily calendar, and also a longer diary for specific days after delivery.

Beyond audit there is the possibility of evaluation. Do the different patterns of care affect differently the health of mothers and babies? This question is far more difficult to answer, because it requires an experimental design such as a randomized controlled trial, and because postnatal care is complex both in its content and its objectives. It is difficult to design a sensible trial that compares, say, a policy of flexible postnatal care agreed between the midwife and the mother with a policy of selective visits in a structured pattern (e.g. day 6, day 8, day 10). This difficulty is due in part to the problem of finding clear objectives for postnatal care. One way to approach the evaluation of postnatal care would be to pick out a group of women with special needs and then test a hypothesis about the content or the pattern of their care. For example, if women at increased risk of postnatal depression were offered midwifery care at home that provided more continuity or that included a structured programme of visits beyond the 10th day, would they do better than if they received standard care?

CONCLUSIONS

Future audit and research in this area will continue to be of great benefit to women and babies. The detailed clinical contents of care need to be described and assessed and the various possible patterns of care audited. More work is needed in order to apply midwifery care appropriately in the postnatal period. While the whole package may not be required for all new mothers, we have to test out effective ways of reaching women with the care that they need. The wider supportive and health promotional elements of the midwife's role should be part of the picture, and the overlapping responsibilities of midwives and health visitors should continue to be explored. We hope that our work in this area will promote more discussion about the best use of midwifery skills in the care of newly delivered women at home.

We are grateful for the contributions of mothers, midwives and colleagues. Funding came from the Wolfson Foundation and the Department of Health.

REFERENCES

ACOG Technical Bulletin (1990) Diagnosis and management of postpartum haemorrhage, *International Journal of Gynaecology and Obstetrics* **36:** 159–63.

Bennett, V.R. and Brown, L.K. (eds) (1993) *Myles Textbook for Midwives*, 12th edn, Edinburgh: Churchill Livingstone.

Central Midwives' Board (1919) *Handbook Incorporating the Rules of the CMB*, 5th edn, London: CMB.

Central Midwives' Board (1935) *Handbook Incorporating the Rules of the CMB*. 12th edn, London: CMB.

Central Midwives' Board (1952) *Handbook Incorporating the Rules of the CMB*. 20th edn, London: CMB.

Central Midwives' Board (1978) *Handbook Incorporating the Rules of the CMB*. *Midwives Rules*. Norwich: Hymns Ancient and Modern Ltd.

Clayton, G. (1987) Beliefs and behaviours. Why is it so hard to change? *Nursing* **3:** 670–3.

Donnison, J. (1988) *Midwives and Medical Men*, London: Historical Publications.

Garcia, J. (1989) *Getting Consumers' Views of Maternity Care: Examples of How the OPCS Survey Manual Can Help*, London: Department of Health.

Garcia, J. and Marchant, S. (1992) *The NPEU Postnatal Care Project*, Research and the Midwife Conference Proceedings. University of Manchester.

Garcia, J., Renfrew, M. and Marchant, S. (1994) Postnatal home visiting by midwives, *Midwifery* **10:** 40–3.

Garforth, S. and Garcia, J. (1989) Hospital admission practices. In Chalmers, I., Enkin, M. and Keirse, M.J.N.C. (eds) *Effective Care in Pregnancy and Childbirth*, pp. 820–6, Oxford: Oxford University Press.

Glazener, C., MacArthur, C. and Garcia, J. (1993) Postnatal care: time for a change. *Contemporary Reviews in Obstetrics and Gynaecology* **5:** 130–6.

Green, J., Coupland, V. and Kitzinger, J. (1988) *Great Expectations: A Prospective Study of Women's Expectations and Experiences of Childbirth*, Cambridge: Child Care and Development Group.

Hall, M., Macintyre, S. and Porter, M. (1985) *Antenatal Care Assessed*, Aberdeen: Aberdeen University Press.

Holden, J.M. (1990) Emotional problems associated with childbirth. In Alexander, A., Levy, V. and Roch, S. (eds) *Postnatal Care – A Research Based Approach*, London: Macmillan.

Holden, J.M., Sagovsky, R. and Cox, L.J. (1989) Counselling in a general practice setting: a controlled study of health visitor intervention in the treatment of postnatal depression, *British Medical Journal* **298:** 223–6.

Hodnett, E. (1994) Support from caregivers during childbirth. In Enkin, M.W., Keirse, M.J.N.C., Renfrew, M.J. and Nielson, J.P. (eds), *Cochrane Collaboration Pregnancy and Childbirth Database*, review No. 03871. Oxford: Update Software.

Loudon, I. (1986) Obstetric care, social class, and maternal mortality, *British Medical Journal* **293:** 606–8.

MacArthur, C., Lewis, M. and Knox, E.G. (1991) *Health After Childbirth*, London: HMSO.

Montgomery, E. and Alexander, J. (1994) Assessing postnatal uterine involution: a review and a challenge, *Midwifery* **10:** 73–6.

Murphy-Black, T. (1989) *Postnatal Care at Home: A Descriptive Study of Mothers' Needs and the Maternity Services. A Report to the Scottish Home and Health Department*, University of Edinburgh, Nursing Research Unit.

Norr, K. and Nacion, K. (1987) Outcomes of postpartum early discharge 1960–1986, *Birth* **14:** 135–41.

Report of the Confidential Enquiry into Maternal Deaths in the United Kingdom (1988–90). London: HMSO.

Robinson, S., Golden, J. and Bradley, S. (1983) The role of the midwife in the provision of postnatal care. In *A Study of the Role and Responsibilities of the Midwife*, Chapter 7, pp. 215–252. Nursing Education Research Unit, Chelsea College, London.

Sleep, J. (1991) Perineal care: a series of five randomised controlled trials. In Robinson, S. and Thomson, A. (eds) *Midwives, Research and Childbirth*, Vol. 2, pp. 199–251, London: Chapman & Hall.

Twaddle, S., Liao, X. and Fyvie, H. (1993) An evaluation of postnatal care individualised to the needs of the woman, *Midwifery* **9:** 154–60.

UKCC (1986, 1993 and 1994) *The Midwife's Code of Practice*. London: United Kingdom Central Council for Nursing, Midwifery and Health Visiting.

UKCC (1992) *Registrar's Letter. Community postnatal visiting by midwives*. London: United Kingdom Central Council for Nursing, Midwifery and Health Visiting.

Walsh, M. and Ford, P. (1989) *Making Observations in Nursing Rituals*, pp. 50–61. Oxford: Heineman Nursing.

White, A., Freeth, S. and O'Brien, M. (1992) *Infant Feeding 1990*, London: Social Survey Division, Office of Population Censuses and Surveys.

5

Educating for the Future

Louise Silverton

INTRODUCTION

Midwifery and midwifery education are in a state of change. The introduction of the purchaser–provider split for both health provision and education has had huge implications for midwifery practice and therefore for all aspects of midwifery education. In addition, the Health Select Committee Report (1992) and Government responses to it will have huge implications for both the preparation and continuing education of midwives. Questions that will need to be answered include what sort of preparation will be required for the midwife of the future, how can midwives keep their knowledge and skills up to date, how may midwifery education be provided, and what will be the contribution of midwives to the education and training of other members of the health care team? This chapter will explore these issues.

WHITHER MIDWIFERY EDUCATION?

Midwifery education has in recent years undergone major changes. Most notable are those relating to the geographical location, the lines of accountability and the financing of midwifery education. Previously in England and Wales, education was considered to be an adjunct of the midwifery service with the school being sited in the maternity unit and the salaries of teachers and students being administered via the midwifery budget by the head of midwifery services (this was sometimes devolved to the senior midwife teacher who also held the position of Approved Midwife Teacher). (Scotland has had combined Colleges of Nursing and Midwifery since 1977 and some of the issues discussed here do not apply in that country.) There were advantages and disadvantages to this situation. One strength was that the geographical proximity of school and clinical area facilitated close links between education and service. Also there were few philosophical differences between the head of the school and the head of service as to the purpose and importance of education for midwives as professionals distinct from nurses. A disadvantage was that the small size of the schools meant that educational infrastructure such as libraries and audio-visual services could be limited, teachers worked in small groups, which was not always cost effective, nor did the small size encourage easy exchange of ideas within a wider educational arena. Finally there were instances where increasing demands upon the midwifery service resulted in cuts in the funding of education which was not always separately identified. Graduate status for midwife teachers was hard to achieve as funding was very limited and also it was hard to release staff from an already small team.

The next change that occurred from the mid to late 1980s was the amalgamation of schools of midwifery to become a college of midwifery or, in most cases, with schools of nursing to become a college of nursing and midwifery or of health. In some areas there have been two or even three different amalgamations to create even larger institutions. The establishment of colleges of midwifery enhanced the autonomous nature of midwifery education, allowed interchange of ideas amongst midwife teachers and has produced economies of scale. Unfortunately none of these colleges has been allowed to survive because some Regional Health Authorities (who were the educational commissioners in England) did not understand the discrete nature of midwifery and were mainly interested in large, all-encompassing institutions. (It is hardly likely that a similar situation would have been imposed upon a school of medicine and dentistry with each profession not having at the very least a separate faculty.) The large midwifery colleges formed in the Birmingham and Manchester areas have linked with colleges of nursing with all the attendant problems of such an arrangement.

The linking that occurred with schools of nursing was not always to the advantage of midwifery with its small numbers of both students and teachers. In some cases, midwifery was viewed as just another branch or specialism of nursing, as happened in Scotland with the head of midwifery education being employed on a similar grade to the leader of children's nursing. Indeed, some midwifery senior tutors found themselves responsible to a nurse educator rather than directly to the college principal, and midwife teachers were not always eligible to apply for senior positions within the institutions (Warwick 1992). Midwife teachers often found themselves often geographically isolated either from midwifery practice areas and or from the wider college. This does not assist with the maintenance of clinical links or with integration with other constituent parts of the college. Midwife teachers are constantly having to explain how midwifery is different from nursing and how arrangements that were satisfactory for the former may not suit the latter (Warwick 1992). One advantage of the move into a larger institution was that services available on a larger scale, such as a well-equipped wide-ranging library, recruitment departments, information technology and specialist academic subject lecturers, were now available for use by midwifery students and their teachers. In addition funding was removed from the midwifery budget (by top slicing) and was administered by Regional Health Authorities in England and on a national basis elsewhere. However, the Approved Midwife Teacher was not always in control of her own budget, a recommendation of the Select Committee Report (1992). Once top slicing to pay for the preparation of future trained staff members became explicit, some service providers began to examine very carefully their need for newly qualified staff. They had the aim of reducing projected levels of recruitment and reclaiming some of the training monies. This has also been accompanied by exercises in skill mix (again financially driven) which in many cases has led to a reduction in the proportion and/or the actual number of trained professionals employed. At the same time as the basis on which the requirements for newly qualified staff are calculated has altered, there has been a reduction in the numbers of both students taught and teachers employed.

The next move that has not yet happened in all areas has been the move into higher education. Links with higher education have been in place for some time now with courses leading to a registerable qualification being jointly validated by the National Board for Nurses, Midwives and Health Visitors and an institution of higher education. For the most part, once midwifery educators became aware of the differing priorities of both parties in the validation process; the Statutory Body being concerned mainly with knowledge, clinical practice and competence whilst higher education is concerned primarily with academic standards; there were few difficulties.

Much more problematic, however, has been the physical and intellectual move into higher education. This, in some cases, has seen midwifery being further marginalized because of its small size. The ideal solution of midwifery achieving its own educational sub-unit (for example as a school within a faculty of health studies) has rarely been achieved (Warwick 1992) perhaps as a result of the small size and the perceived limited importance of midwifery education in the Health Service. Significantly higher administration costs in higher education (including overheads and employers' pension contributions) has meant a reduction in numbers of teachers employed. The need for all teachers to be graduates (rather than to be studying for a degree) has sometimes disadvantaged midwives who, because of lack of financial assistance and their smaller numbers (than nurse teachers), have been later in achieving their degrees. (This has been especially problematic where the teachers are moving into a traditional university.) The geographical isolation of teaching sites from practice areas has reduced opportunities for clinical teaching and contacts between teachers and midwives. This may in turn further threaten the practice base of midwifery education programmes. This split from practice has been accentuated by the fact that most clinical areas now have Trust status whilst the midwife teachers are either employees of a directly managed unit within the Health Service or of an institute of higher education. This leads to problems negotiating clinical placements for students and the loss of the mutually beneficial relationship where education and service could help each other. Where there is poor understanding of the nature of midwifery, clinical teaching may not be valued by the higher education establishment and teachers discouraged from spending time in practice areas. In addition, in order to reduce costs, shared learning of key academic disciplines with other students may be imposed. Where this is a variance with the needs of the curriculum and course philosophy it has been shown to be counter productive (Kent *et al.* 1994).

One must ask what is the future for midwifery education? Have the changes gone too far so that the profession is now seen as a minor branch of nursing? How can midwifery educators fight back to regain their direct lines of communication within the hierarchy? These issues were considered by the Royal College of Midwives (RCM) in their document, *Guidelines for the Provision of Midwifery Education* (1993) (to be revised in 1996). In it they have documented where statements from the Statutory Bodies, the Department of Health or other authorities have pointed out the discrete and separate nature of midwifery education. Included in this is the statement that the structure of the institution must take account of the uniqueness of midwifery, the position and status of the head of midwifery education must be acknowledged, the need for budgetary control to be in the hands of the head of midwifery education and that she also has control over the midwifery education strategy and the curriculum. This is an issue also considered by the Select Committee in their report (1992, para 417) which said:

> *We recommend that midwives should be afforded the same rights as all other professions over the control of their education. Midwifery studies should be accorded independent faculty status. Selection of candidates, curriculum planning, assessment processes and course validation must remain under the control of the midwifery profession. We would expect these principles to be upheld not only in the training establishments but also by the statutory bodies.*
>
> (Select Committee 1992, p. xxxvi)

In order for the RCM document (1993) to have any strength it must be used by midwife teachers and its contents raised in discussion with the Statutory Body in order to avoid approval of structures, policies or curriculums that are contrary to the interests of midwifery. It is also necessary for midwifery educators to speak out; although we are few in number compared with nurses we are often well advanced in the areas of curriculum design, assessment of clinical practice, education/service links and involvement in all levels of teaching (basic and ongoing). Not only can we learn from nursing but they have much to learn from us. We must not be scared or shy of contributing our experiences.

The continuing threat to midwifery control of its education has been compounded by the position allotted to the senior midwifery educator within the academic hierarchy. She is frequently not a part of the faculty of college management team and is denied the opportunity to influence policy at an appropriate level. In Scotland a report into nursing and midwifery education (Scottish Office 1994) followed a nursing model that took no account of the different nature of midwifery education. Senior midwifery educators in Scotland are often placed at the same level in the hierarchy as those who lead the smaller branches of nursing and cannot therefore influence the process. The Scottish Office Report (1994) appears to be based solely on reducing the cost of student bursaries with grants and loans than by any financial or educational consideration. The recent recommendation by the English National Board (ENB 1994, currently being deferred) to remove the recommended teacher–student ratios will make it much easier for establishments to employ non–midwife teachers to teach midwives than at present. It also puts under threat the clinical commitment of those teachers, especially now that they have the additional need to demonstrate that they are actively involved in research.

EDUCATION FOR REGISTRATION

All midwifery education has as its minimum end-point the United Kingdom Central Council (UKCC) and European Union midwifery competencies (UKCC 1991). Whilst much debate has surrounded the best way of achieving these competencies, what has not been questioned is 'What type of practice are we preparing midwives for?' For example, previously, the philosophy of the educational programme or institution was often not considered (Bennett 1988) but now it must be explicit if all involved with the programme are to act in unison. (Where the philosophy is known the imposition of shared learning with professions with varying philosophies is even less educationally sound.) Within the profession there has been a move for midwives to reclaim their role, giving total care throughout pregnancy, labour and the puerperium to an identified group of women rather than as happens in many cases to a large number of often unknown women for a short time period or one specific care episode (Robinson 1989a,b). This midwife exercises her full range of skills, liaises with and/or refers to other professional groups as an equal and provides research-based care as the main carer throughout pregnancy, labour and the puerperium

(Select Committee 1992). This so-called 'new midwife' will not become a reality unless the profession is united on what she is and on the best way in which to prepare her (Page 1993). In addition any attempt to produce this new individual will surely falter if the learning environment (either clinical or classroom) is contradictory or hostile to the agreed philosophy of the teachers or leaders of the profession.

This section asks some questions about the type of preparation we are giving to new practitioners and whether the spur to change has been the well-being of women and children or financial and government-led expediency.

The most appropriate route

The introduction of more readily accessible three-year pre-registration midwifery preparation has yet to be evaluated fully. (The report of the implementation of the programmes is available (Kent *et al.* 1994) but the review of outcomes is ongoing.) Its recent resurgence came about as a result of an anticipated future shortage of potential recruits into midwifery from nursing as a result of a decline in the number of 18 year olds in the population eligible and wanting to enter nursing together with reports from schools of midwifery that there was a demand for such education (Bluff 1990). This was combined with a change to diploma level educational programmes (in both midwifery and nursing) to attract school leavers with five GCSEs in competition with other careers such as banking. In reality, however, the economic recession and a reduction in the number of student nurses in training has meant that there is still an oversupply of suitable candidates for nursing. Similarly, reduced mobility of qualified nurses (who form the entrants to the pre-registration (shortened) programme) and a shortage of positions for the newly qualified together with a reduction in midwifery intakes has maintained the waiting list amongst nurses for midwifery education programmes.

The advent of the pre-registration student has created a challenge for teacher and midwife alike (Kent *et al.* 1994) For the teacher, the students have not yet been socialized into the role of a health professional. Students with diverse backgrounds and varied experiences need to quickly grasp the concept of confidentiality and also to adapt to the irregular hours worked by midwives. Teachers have to demonstrate and develop in students the model of what it is to be a professional midwife without suppressing motivation or imposing a nursing model.

Additional issues of pre-registration preparation have centred around the organization of the curriculum. The competencies to be achieved are clearly laid down by the UKCC (1991) and the European Union but there is much freedom in the order and method by which they are reached and also when considering any additional or further knowledge that is given. The simple solution of teaching underlying academic disciplines first has not been universally successful as students cannot always appreciate their relevance and they want to learn about midwifery (Kent *et al.* 1994). However, it is hard for the student to understand, for example, the physiological processes of pregnancy without a background knowledge of the physiology of the non-pregnant woman. When providing clinical teaching and support in the clinical area, there are similar challenges to be overcome. For example, the student must be assisted to make sense of clinical practice without the underlying knowledge. Broad concepts relating, for example, to the aims of antenatal care will need to be used until the student has the knowledge to understand the processes in more detail. An additional issue is that midwives are used to teaching and supervising students who have basic nursing skills; not only do these need to be taught and practised but the student must also be able to contribute to the care given in a meaningful manner. Although the students are supernumerary for the first 2 years of their programme, it is only through hands-on experience that they will learn. Limiting access to the clinical setting in the first year to allow time for classroom work can only affect motivation leading to possible dropping out of the course for unhappy students who expected a more practical inclination (Kent *et al.* 1994). Several compromises have been developed that suit local areas. These include limiting the observation of practice in the early months to allow basic and midwifery theory to be studied concurrently. None is ideal.

The current situation where the vast majority of midwives have entered the profession via nursing may, in the future, be seen as an anachronism. In many countries midwifery and nursing are two separate professions with no reduction in training for an individual qualified in either of them (World Health Organization (WHO) 1985). Midwives with no other qualification cannot practice as nurses if jobs are scarce or satisfaction is low; it is up to the profession to ensure that only enough midwives as are required are trained. This will give the professional a scarcity value which may help in the fight for appropriate pay. An ongoing project to ensure that Scotland, Wales and Northern Ireland and each Region in England are self-sufficient in trained midwives is aimed at preventing under- or over-training. (This is known in England as the National Balance Sheet.) However, before the level of education commissions can be decided upon there needs to be an accurate projection of future workforce needs. The previous lack of any national coordination of workforce planning has meant that the tool has had to be developed from scratch. This exercise depends on locally obtained information as to the projected number of staff leaving or retiring, determination of future levels of work load (such as new methods of care provision) and inputs from the private and voluntary sector. This model has many potential sources of error which, if compounded, could lead to massive under- or over-training. Since the first three rounds of this exercise have all led to significant reduction in the numbers of student mid-wives recruited (together with a loss of midwifery education posts), it is hard to see the latter occurring. It appears from figures from the third round of the process that there may be a shortage of newly trained staff in 1997/8.

One side-effect of the current financial situation in the health service with its reduction in the numbers of midwives in training may be a future shortage of midwives. These cutbacks are often due to a shortage of money or a decrease in current demands for midwives (due to increased retention or cuts in estab-lishment); an increased need in the future may not be able to be met if the mid-wife teachers and clinical support staff are no longer there. The profession must also be wary of a reduction in midwifery numbers as cheaper alternatives may be suggested or aspects of care central to the midwives' role may be given to another professional. This has happened in Germany where most antenatal care is given by doctors and postnatal care by nurses with midwives only giving care in labour (WHO 1985). Another issue central to retention within the profes-sion is the ensuring of adequate career progression (this includes a different and less hierarchical career structure from that used by nurses) one of the keys to which is continuing education (see below). (Midwifery lends itself to a more flattened career structure than does nursing with each midwife carrying her own or sharing a defined case load.) There must no discrimination against the non-nurse midwife with all positions requiring a midwifery qualification being open to her. It is important that the three-year programme (which is a quicker and cheaper option than the post-nursing route) is not simply supported for financial reasons and also is not undervalued thus disadvantaging its diplomates (Radford and Thompson 1988).

An important aspect of pre-registration education is that of shared learning. This has proved a contentious point amongst both midwives and nurses. Shared learning can be applied on two levels: similar level students from dif-ferent professions studying together or mixing qualified and unqualified mem-bers of the same profession. I would argue that there is only one instance in which shared learning is fully acceptable and one where it is partly so. The former is where experienced staff can learn from the application of basic and common elements (such as research methodology) to the work of other pro-fessional groups as in continuing education for nurses, midwives and health visitors or in the preparation for teachers to many different professional groups. These sessions should be followed by seminars and tutorials particular to the profession which examine specific applications of the theory. Such an approach must also be used where student and qualified midwives learn together. I would argue that this is only appropriate for keynote lectures, i.e. those concerned with pure information giving. Any discussion or further study should separate the two groups. Where ongoing professional education is concerned, evaluations from shared conferences with midwives, general practitioners (GPs) and obstetricians indicate that this is a good format for discussing practice issues.

Contrary to the opinion of some midwifery educators (Ho 1990) I would oppose the sharing of learning between pre-registration students in midwifery and nursing. My argument here is that the student midwives are usually outnumbered, may not yet have a clear idea of their professional identity and because of this the nursing bias that is frequently presented causes the midwifery students to become dissociated from, or dissatisfied with, the subject matter. Indeed, Kent *et al.* (1994) have shown that shared learning, far from highlighting similarities between groups of students, serves mainly to demonstrate differences and is often seen as irrelevant. Jackson (1993) is also against shared learning for student midwives and nurses but for different reasons. She argues that the need for the midwife teacher to highlight the relevance of information in shared sessions is repeating the worst aspects of midwifery education programmes of the past with their statutory obstetrics lectures. In addition shared learning can lead to midwives losing control of the midwifery curriculum. Shared learning for student midwives is often introduced to reduce the costs of lectures for the supporting academic disciplines. This is not an appropriate rationale. If midwives need this knowledge (and I am not always convinced that at such an early stage they do), then they have a right to have it applied to their area of practice from the start and not as an afterthought.

The required academic level?

The move, over the past decade, to raise the academic status of midwifery preparation has, to a major extent, been unquestioned. This is surprising because midwifery is such a practical profession and one where status should not depend solely on academic achievement (Jackson 1993). It has been viewed that education is a 'good thing', therefore more education is better. If this rise in academic level is simply to counter the position of medical staff then I would argue that this is an inappropriate reason. If it was to improve the care given to mothers and babies by developing critical and analytical thinking (Page and Healey 1990), whatever the effects in other areas, then this is the only appropriate rationale.

The introduction of Diploma level preparation (to provide academic status and therefore attract people into midwifery; one must ask are these the right sort of people?) has been seen by many practitioners and midwifery educators as only an interim step before all midwives are prepared to degree level. Two related questions must then be answered: firstly, what is the effect on midwifery care of these changes; and secondly, are we undervaluing the study of midwifery by such a concentration on the underlying academic disciplines (Jackson

1993)? It is already known that some women are alienated from their doctors by the latter's educational level and social class. Will we, by aligning ourselves so closely with higher education, be denying entry to the profession to those who do not have or have not had the opportunity to gain the required entry qualifications? Will we be creating a midwifery elite rather than preparing the midwife to be 'with woman'? This is not to argue against midwives being graduates but to suggest that for many this is a status that they should perhaps gain when they have sufficient professional experience. Empirical evidence shows that when the use and comprehension of midwifery issues are compared between a newly qualified diploma midwife and one of some experience who has studied the Diploma in Professional Studies in Midwifery, the latter is, as would be expected, more rooted in practice and better able to use her new knowledge. Perhaps a compromise will be reached by giving the new entrant to the profession the introductory knowledge required to achieve competence but following this with a structured programme over the 2 or 3 years following registration? This would have the added advantage of not barring from entry to the profession older women or those denied access to, or success in, traditional educational programmes.

The position of students within the new health service

Students enrich the clinical environment by prompting staff to question their own actions and to act as models of good practice. It is known from nursing that areas without students can stagnate clinically or can lose those staff who miss the challenge of practice development and the presence of an inquiring mind. Removing learners from areas of poor clinical practice protects the learners but does not improve the environment for those receiving care. However, having students present in clinical practice puts a financial burden on the area as it may take the professional longer to perform her duties whilst she is instructing or supervising learners. The principle of payment for access to clinical areas has already been accepted in some settings and may soon enter midwifery. A possible solution to this problem is either to provide the clinical support for students from the educational institution (see below) or to give back something to the practice area in return such as continuing education for the qualified staff. Indeed, some educational contracts specify the existence of this 'added value' factor.

The advent of supernumerary status for students together with the use of clinical staff as mentors or preceptors has opened up the debate regarding the position of students as apprentices. (The term apprentice, although originally meaning a person working under legal agreement for a specified time for a master craftsman is now used to describe someone learning a craft or trade under particular conditions.)

Traditionally in midwifery this term has been used for the learning undertaken by lay or traditional midwives (Gaskin 1991). It exists in the USA for both indigenous and licensed midwives such as those prepared by the Seattle midwifery school (Silverton 1988, Myers-Ciecko 1991). The concept of apprenticeship could indeed be easily adopted for British midwives with students being attached for most of their experience to one midwifery team. This would have several advantages; students would have access to the full range of midwifery practice whilst giving care to a defined group of women, thus stressing the importance of childbearing as a continuing process rather than isolated events. Thus the student could be prepared within a model of midwifery practice envisaged by the Select Committee Report (1992). The student would be exposed to fewer midwives than now as role models but she would have some choice in the event of a personality clash and the midwives themselves would see the student as a member of the team to be nurtured and supported rather than as a transient guest or interloper. The use of a team of midwives to teach the student would mean that the roles of preceptor and assessor for any stage of the preparation could be separated, thus reducing a potential conflict.

The learning environment

It is well known from both nursing and midwifery education that a gap between theory and practice creates conflict and unhappiness amongst students. Development of clinical practice is just as important as the design of the new curriculum (Page and Healey 1990). Educational audit of clinical areas has been introduced to ensure that standards of practice are up to date and in accordance with what is required by the Statutory Body. There is, however, no comparable audit of the classroom as a learning environment or whether the curriculum is being delivered in the spirit within which it was designed. Annual reviews of educational establishments and their associated clinical areas provide only a snapshot of what is going on. Both sides in the educational process need to be committed to the philosophy of the programme with staff being fully prepared and supported in their role, wherever that may be.

Conflict between the holistic nature of midwifery practice as espoused by the curriculum and the medically led care in some consultant obstetric units has led to a change in the way in which practical experience has been gained. The most obvious sign of this has been the move to begin the programme with observational experience in the community where normal family centred care is more likely to be seen. However, the student must at some time be exposed to the hospital environment with its artificial boundaries between areas of care. The question to be posed is how can students develop as autonomous confident midwives when some or much of their practical experience occurs in areas where midwives function as obstetric nurses? The use of lecturer practitioners is one solution but in the current climate they cannot be with the student all of the time. Another solution is the allocation of students to teams of midwives so that they can see the entirety of the role, albeit in different individuals (see earlier).

Preparing a student midwife to meet the demands of the Select Committee Report (1992) or the Government response (Department of Health 1993) cannot occur without a fundamental change in practice. One aspect of the training of GPs that has always been criticized is the fact that most or all of their obstetric experience is hospital based and concerned with the care not of the normal woman, but of those with a high risk of complications (Smith 1990). Is it any wonder then that they are reluctant to support birth at home? This exposure to inappropriate models of midwifery practice should be avoided if at all possible. Few midwifery students currently have the opportunity to be present at a home birth; how will they cope when qualified? Steps must be taken to ensure that all newly qualified midwives have experienced a home birth, even if this means that intake sizes are reduced in the interim period whilst the recommendations of *Changing Childbirth* (Department of Health 1993) are implemented. Additionally, those midwives currently in practice must be supported and encouraged to rediscover or develop the knowledge and skills to equip them to practise as envisaged by the Select Committee Report (1992).

It would be encouraging for those currently seeking to re-establish midwifery as a profession independent of nursing if, in future, entry to the profession is primarily via a 3-year programme to diploma level with a recognized pathway to first and second degree level for experienced midwives. This can only occur if we can show that specialization matters and we resist the move towards genericism already apparent in nursing. It is important to demonstrate that highly educated (that is with both skills and knowledge) midwives produce better care for mothers and babies at no more cost than other care given.

CONTINUING EDUCATION

The history of continuing education in midwifery is one where new programmes are introduced and then whither away or are totally replanned as they outgrow their usefulness. (Many of these developments have been either initiated or advanced by the Royal College of Midwives.) To some extent this is true both of the traditional 5–day midwifery refresher course programme and of the Advanced Diploma in Midwifery, which has been superseded by the Diploma in Professional Studies in Midwifery and latterly by bachelor's and master's level programmes. Continuing education is vital to any profession if its members are not to become set in their ways and unresponsive to the needs of those they serve. This is especially true in midwifery where, as Hunt (1991) argues, it is every woman's right to be cared for by a midwife who is fully up to date with developments in, and issues relating to, her practice. It has been shown that there is often an unmet demand for educational provision which surfaces when there are new initiatives in practice or education (Page and Healey 1990). The expansion of continuing education programmes and their increasing availability locally (some are offered through distance learning) has resulted in many more midwives wanting to study.

This section will look at the provision of continuing education for midwives, including the role of the refresher courses and the type of learning that occurs.

Individual responsibility for knowledge

The UKCC's Code of Professional Conduct states that it is the duty of every professional to keep themselves up to date:

> *As a registered nurse, midwife or health visitor, you are personally accountable for your own practice and, in the exercise of professional accountability, must: maintain and improve professional knowledge and competence and acknowledge any limitations in your knowledge and competence and decline any duties or responsibilities unless able to perform them in a safe and skilled manner.*
>
> (UKCC 1992)

This means that each midwife should remain aware of developments within the profession and regularly update herself as regards new knowledge. As Hunt (1991) states, the practitioner is not allowed to stand still but she must 'move forwards, onwards and upwards'. However, traditional methods of teaching did not always foster such self-analysis nor did they give the individual the skills necessary to assess their own needs, especially if she was unaware of any deficiencies. The profession has relied on mandatory periodic refreshment plus the assessment of the supervisor of midwives of any defect in knowledge or skills to identify and meet continuing education needs. Whilst of practical use, deficits in skills and/or knowledge were often gross before they were detected. The UKCC's (1994) requirements under PREP (Post Registration, Education and Practice) will require each practitioner to demonstrate that their chosen activities of continuing professional development have maintained their competence to practice.

The current development of unitized diploma, undergraduate and post-graduate programmes for midwives has increased both the range and accessibility of educational provision. Midwives who have not studied for some time are often reticent about putting themselves forward for these courses and they may benefit from some return-to-study programmes to raise self-confidence. These can also incorporate skills such as profiling which will help the midwife to assess what it is she wants to achieve and also what skills and knowledge are already in her possession. The use of both accreditation of prior experiential learning (APEL) and accreditation of prior learning (APL) will do much to give midwives a feeling of self-worth and to show them how much they have learnt in the time since qualification.

Periodic refreshment

Statutory refresher courses for midwives (1 week every 5 years for those in practice and return-to-practice programmes for those who are not) were laid down by the 1936 Midwives' Act. The courses were not established until after the Second World War. The original courses were planned as a 5-day programme of lectures usually as a residential programme. Many midwives attended each course (sometimes in excess of 150) and it is only from the mid 1980s that the courses developed a more explicit educational bias with smaller numbers of attendees (50–80), specialist themes for the week, the use of group work and discussions assisted by facilitators.

Little authoritative work has been carried out as to the value of these 1-week old format courses. This could be because, as the author herself discovered, the measurement tool was too complex to develop and validate. Whilst one could simply assess new knowledge gained, the effect, if any, of this on the midwife's practice or her attitudes was almost unmeasurable. Asking a Supervisor of Midwives to comment on an individual's performance was felt to be too intrusive, ethically unsound and too subjective to permit easy comparison. The midwife's own assessment of the value of the programme often had more to do with the setting, catering arrangements and type of fellow midwives on the course than its educational value. It is perhaps for these reasons that most research relating to refreshment programmes has examined the process and content rather than the outcomes.

The change to accumulated refresher days, which began in England in the late 1980s and has since been followed by Scotland and Northern Ireland, was welcomed by midwives and their managers, the latter perhaps because of a reduction in financial outlay and greater flexibility of timing. (Previous residential courses were often held in university accommodation and therefore tended to take place in peak holiday periods over Easter and in the summer.) The rationale behind the change was that the effectiveness of the 5-day residential programmes was in doubt: they were geared towards the mass rather than the individual. Also, as more midwives have young children or are in part-time employment, the traditional courses were less convenient. Short courses of one or a few days allow coverage of a smaller range of subjects which can be considered in greater depth.

Theoretically the accumulated days would better facilitate the midwife to update herself. This may involve guidance and discussion from her supervisor in assisting her to choose attendance at those sessions of greatest relevance. However, the accumulated days have yet to be evaluated (other than their acceptability to the midwife at the time) and there is a tendency for attendance to be due to the convenience of the midwifery service as regards timing or location rather than to the subject matter of the day. By using her professional profile as laid down by PREP (UKCC 1994), the midwife will need to show how her learning needs have been met by the activities undertaken. This should ensure a better match than occurs at present. Some midwives may require initial assistance with assessing their learning needs and evaluating which activities will best meet their individual requirements. They will also need to balance work and other commitments with their choice of activity. For some, certain methods such as open learning may be inappropriate, for example where family commitments do not permit quiet study. For this reason some midwives may still decide to undertake one of the new 5-day refresher programmes as a part of their continuing development. However, once these programmes are no longer required to meet the continuing education needs of the mass of midwives they can be focused on particular subject areas.

In recent years there has been a widening of the type of educational programme, attendance at which can be used as an alternative to a traditional refresher course. These have included many of the units and modules designed specifically for midwives in the various continuing education programmes offered in each of the four home countries. This expansion in educational provision which is recognized for refreshment purposes has had the effect of allowing motivated midwives not to have to do extra study on top of what they are already doing. It has also encouraged some others to broaden their horizons from the traditional 5-day programme and to consider less structured forms of study. It remains to be seen how far this will go towards fostering the life-long habit of learning required of a professional and also by PREP (UKCC 1994).

Education for change

The NHS has recently found itself in a climate of almost perpetual change. For many employees this is very stressful; the lower the position of the individual in the hierarchy, the greater the level of stress (Lazarus 1966). In addition, in order to make the best of change imposed from on high, midwives are themselves trying to introduce change. For example, midwives in England are currently using the recommendations contained in *Changing Childbirth* (Department of Health 1993) to propose innovations in their management of care that will help them to fulfil their role. To that end, midwives need the knowledge and skills both to respond to and implement change. I would argue that all midwives need to know how best to respond to change whilst the change agents within the profession should be identified, prepared and encouraged in their role. A knowledge of the change process would assist midwives to adopt the role of change agent and would help others to see their role in the achievement of change.

The current climate of almost perpetual change within health care makes it vital that midwives can respond quickly to new initiatives and also propose and implement novel solutions. For some midwives they may need to gain new skills together with advancing their knowledge. For others, all that may be required is the fostering of a belief in themselves and a raising of professional esteem which may have faltered after years of struggle with other professions and with officialdom. When midwives are regarded as purely specialist nurses and are treated as such, it is all too easy to believe in the brain-washing. This is especially true in high dependency or medically led units where child-bearing women are referred to and treated as patients and midwives are employed to work within a hierarchy that fosters obedience and routines whilst discouraging professional independence and individual autonomy. This last situation can create severe conflict for the midwife who lacks either the skills (such as assertiveness) or knowledge to deal with it, especially when she remains professionally accountable for all her actions and inactions.

Adult learning

The concept of adult learning has been adopted by most midwifery educators for both education leading to registration as a midwife and for continuing education. This concept means that the student takes responsibility for her own learning with the support and guidance of a teacher. Students are very much a part of the learning process contributing to it with their experiences. In adult learning, within the parameters of the programme (especially where it involves a recordable or registerable qualification), students can decide how the end-point can best be reached. This can include both the course content and its mode of delivery. These are then negotiated with and agreed by the programme leader.

A central part of adult learning in midwifery is the use of learning contracts. These can be drawn up on an individual or group basis and are agreed by the teacher and student(s). Individual contracts permit the student or midwife to set their own goals with points of achievement along the way. There is agreement as to how much and what sort of study will be undertaken as well as how and when the advice and support of the teacher will be sought. Taking responsibility for one's own learning is important for the whole area of professional updating and can also assist in raising an individual's assessment of their self-worth. The use of learning contracts should be taught during return-to-study programmes as part of the process of self-assessment as it requires specific skills.

WHO SHOULD EDUCATE MIDWIVES?

The specialist teacher versus the lecturer practitioner

The specialist preparation of teachers of midwives was laid down in the 1936 Midwives' Act. At that time there was no formal preparation for those who taught and/or supported midwives in the classroom or in clinical practice. There have been various changes in the preparation of midwife teachers over the years. Most recently these have included making the Advanced Diploma in Midwifery (now combined with the Diploma in Professional Studies (midwifery)) mandatory before embarking on a teaching course (alternatives are now acceptable), the move from specialist Midwife Teacher's Diploma (MTD) programmes to generalist certificate and Diploma programmes in the education of adults to now ensuring that all new entrants to teaching have at least first degree level qualifications. This is to ensure the academic base of the teacher, to develop the knowledge and also to ensure that they are qualified to at least one level higher than the students they teach (most of whom are on Diploma of Higher Education (Dip HE) programmes). There have been similar changes in clinical areas with midwives being prepared for their role as teacher by undertaking a course on teaching and assessing in clinical practice.

As the classroom side of education has become geographically, and in some cases philosophically, isolated from clinical practice areas, teachers and midwives have tried to close the gap by having link lecturers who liaise with and provide support in a defined area. Where these teachers have regular (usually weekly) and ongoing commitment to midwifery practice, they may be referred to as lecturer practitioners, a term with many diverse meanings. However, this is not always an ideal situation because, where pressures of work intervene, it is usually the classroom aspects of the job that take precedence. This gives the teacher who prefers not to practise an acceptable excuse not to do so; it also disappoints both students and clinical staff who feel that they cannot rely on the teacher and may therefore not encourage the relationship. The English National Board has recognized the importance of clinical practice for all teachers and has recommended that 20% of the teacher's time (1 day per week) is spent in the clinical situation. It is unclear how this ruling will be policed or monitored.

An alternative solution is to examine the whole way in which midwives are taught. It could be argued that now there are specialist subject teachers for those underlying academic disciplines that support midwifery knowledge and practice, there is less need for so many classroom-based full-time midwife teachers. Perhaps resources would be better employed by having two types of midwifery educators? A traditional educator who is mainly classroom-based, with responsibility for curriculum design, assessment, classroom teaching, educational research and a small, clearly defined clinical commitment and a greater number of practice-based teachers who carry their own identified clinical case load, undertake classroom teaching of clinical subjects but do most of their teaching and assessing in practical situations (a model followed by the medical profession). This would then provide the student with an appropriate role model in practice, would reduce any potential gap between theory and practice and could possibly provide a solution (if partly funded by education) to the issue of clinical mangers being reluctant to have students working in their area.

Oxford have created two types of lecturer practitioner: one where the midwife teacher combines her role with that of a senior midwife in a defined clinical area and another where the teaching role is combined with that of being a team leader (Page and Healey 1990). I would, however, recommend caution before following this model as there are risks of overburdening the lecturer practitioner who performs 1.5 or even 2 full-time roles leaving her at risk of burn-out.

Conflict between the roles of mentor and assessor

The definition of a mentor is that of a 'teacher or coach' and that of a preceptor is defined as 'teacher'; thus, if one uses purely a dictionary definition, there is little difference. The use of such terms to describe a practising midwife who teaches and supports students in the clinical situation has allowed one-to-one or one-to-two teaching to be acknowledged. However, the situation can give rise to conflict where the mentor or preceptor is also required to assess her student. It could be argued that the role of assessor is implicit in that of teacher with the converse viewpoint that the term teacher refers to the provider of formal education in the classroom and not to the close relationships formed through clinical practice. Perhaps one solution would be for the initial and interim assessment of the student to be performed by the mentor but for another midwife or a classroom-based teacher to jointly mark the final clinical assessment. Certainly where students have the same midwife as mentor for a long period of time, a close bond can form between the two that may prevent objectivity on behalf of the midwife. In a situation where mentorship is working properly, any problems with the student's performance would have been identified and rectified long before the final summative assessment occurred. The use of educational audit and the role of external examiner can also be used to ensure the validity of a sample of assessments.

Can midwives afford not to teach students?

The role of teacher is implicit within that of the midwife, that is as the teacher of future and new parents. The principles of teaching are included within midwifery education programmes. However, some midwives do not enjoy teaching, feel that they are not equipped for it or are not sufficiently confident in their role to teach others. Because teaching is so central to the midwife's role and because of her duty to practise to the highest possible standards, it could be argued that all midwives should teach both parents and students and that there should be no opportunity to opt out.

With the advent of hospital and community trusts it may be that there are designated teaching midwives as have been used previously in the community or that clinical support will come from midwives employed by the educational institution. This will be a lost opportunity because all midwives should be willing to subject their practice to the scrutiny and enquiring eyes of the student, who can prompt the midwife to question her practice and thus provide further impetus for her to keep up to date. It will also cause those midwives who currently function only as obstetric nurses to feel uncomfortable and perhaps examine the way in which they are not fulfilling their role.

WHO ELSE SHOULD MIDWIVES TEACH?

The role and preparation of the midwifery support worker

Support workers have always existed in some form or another in both nursing and maternity wards. However, the regularizing of their training and role came about as one of the conditions put forward by Central Government for the introduction of the Project 2000 curriculum into nursing. With the reduction of the service contribution made by students, support workers would be introduced to replace them. Also, in addition, the present *ad hoc* system of support worker preparation would be replaced by a scheme overseen by the National Council for Vocational Qualifications. The training programmes would be at various levels of complexity. Should a support worker obtain certain qualifications then she or he would have the entry requirements to commence preparation as a nurse. The introduction of Project 2000, the economic recession and the advent of Trust status within the NHS as a result of the Government White paper 'Working for Patients' has meant that many managers have seen the increased employment of support workers as a means of reducing the total salary bill.

When the organized and coherent strategy for the preparation and employment of support workers was discussed with the midwifery profession it received a lukewarm response. It was envisaged that the only roles suitable would be either secretarial or domestic in nature. However, managers have been increasing the numbers of support workers employed in maternity settings and to this end the profession could be said to have been naive and to have missed a valuable opportunity. Had the support worker concept been embraced earlier, the profession could have had a major influence on their preparation and employment. It is quite possible that there may be a future opportunity for the profession to assist in the preparation of support workers in such a way that these workers can be used to enhance the status of midwives and to improve the total care given to mothers and babies. There are models of this in other countries such as the Maternity Aide in The Netherlands.

In this country the highly trained midwifery support worker could be the second person present during a home birth, could assist with the general care and support of the mother and baby following home birth or early transfer from hospital (especially after an operative birth) and could give support to the breastfeeding mother. All of this would improve the service being offered whilst enhancing rather than diminishing the midwife's role. In light of the recent reports on the future of the maternity services (Department of Health 1993), perhaps now is the time for midwives to be arguing for specially prepared midwifery support workers who could reduce costs of hospital stay by supporting the new mother at home and facilitating maternal choice.

Contribution to the preparation of general practitioners

General practice trainees have traditionally received their preparation for the fields of obstetrics and gynaecology by having a 6–12-month placement in a consultant maternity unit and on gynaecological wards. Recently the inappropriateness of this has been acknowledged, as it introduces trainees to high technology care and the support and surveillance of those at high risk of complications. Smith (1991) has reported that a significant number of those who have undertaken experience in obstetrics prior to entering general practice did not feel competent in normal childbirth. For example, of GPs offering full obstetric care, 37% did not feel competent to undertake a normal delivery unaided, a figure that rose to 54% of those giving shared care. The end result is that the GP, when in practice, may be reluctant to undertake intrapartum care because he or she does not feel comfortable outside the hospital environment or because they feel that childbirth is too risky.

A joint committee of the Royal College of General Practitioners and the Royal College of Obstetricians and Gynaecologists (1993) have reviewed the preparation of GPs in this area. They see a need to stress the normality of most of childbirth and they recommend the use of alternative forms of practical experience such as time spent working with a midwife and community ante-natal clinics. This would have the advantage of removing the fear of childbirth held by some GPs and also allowing them to see the full extent of the midwife's role and responsibilities. Shared learning alongside student midwives and qual-ified staff undergoing updating programmes could occur. The profession must welcome such an initiative and give educational support as required. It has been acknowledged that midwives have a lot to offer in the field of education, not least our experience in teaching and assessing in practice settings.

CONCLUSIONS

Midwifery and, in particular, midwifery education are at a crossroads with two paths, one of which leads to full professional independence and the other to professional demise and oblivion as a branch of nursing. It is up to midwives and midwife teachers to agree which path to take (as if there is any choice), to resist the blandishments of nursing educationists that 'we are all in this together' and to go forward using the current unsettled climate as an opportunity to achieve what we want. That is, independent professional education for mid-wives led by midwife teachers with midwifery at the forefront supported by but not subsumed by the underlying academic disciplines. For this to occur, teachers must stand up for themselves but they must also be supported by mid-wives in practice if they are not to be the end of the breed. The current oppor-tunities given to us by the Select Committee Report (1992) and its governmental interpretations are a once in a lifetime occurrence whose use must not be squandered. If we do so we will bear the discomfort and poor ser-vice given to women and their babies on our consciences.

REFERENCES

Bennett, V.R. (1988) 'Horizons in Midwifery Education', *Midwives Chronicle*, June, pp. 178–81.

Bluff, R. (1990) 'Assessment of Demand for Direct Entry Midwifery Training', *Midwives Chronicle*, August, pp. 238–40.

Department of Health (1993) *Changing Childbirth*, London: HMSO.

English National Board (1994) *Board Decisions Relating to Staff: Student Ratios in Nursing and Midwifery Education* (Ref DCL/24/RLV), London: ENB.

Ho, E. (1990) 'Direct Entry Curriculum Model', *Midwives Chronicle*, August, pp. 242–4.

Hunt, S.C. (1991) 'Continuing Education For Midwives. A Woman's Right', *Midwives Chronicle*, January, pp. 6–7.

Gaskin, I.M. (1991) Midwifery reinvented. In Kitzinger, S. (ed.) *The Midwife Challenge*, 2nd edn, pp. 42–60, London: Pandora.

Jackson, K. (1993) Midwifery degree programmes: who benefits, *British Journal of Midwifery* **1(6):** 274–5.

Kent, J., MacKeith, N. and Maggs, C. (1994) *Direct But Different*, Bath: Maggs Research Associates.

Lazarus, R.S. (1966) *Psychological Stress and the Coping Process*, New York: McGraw Hill.

Myers-Ciecko, J. (1991) Direct entry midwifery in the USA. In Kitzinger, S. (ed.) *The Midwife Challenge,* 2nd edn, pp. 61–86, London: Pandora.

Page, L. (1993) Education for practice, *MIDIRS Midwifery Digest* **3(3):** 253–6.

Page, L. and Healey, E. (1990) Midwifery by degree: changes in education and service in Oxford, *Midwife, Health Visitor and Community Nurse* **26(10):** 365.

Radford, N. and Thompson, A. (1988) 'Choosing the Design', *Nursing Times*, Vol. 84, No. 32, pp. 42–3.

Robinson, S. (1989a) Caring for childbearing woman: the inter-relationship between midwifery and medical responsibilities. In Robinson, S. and Thomson, A.M. (eds) *Midwives, Research and Childbirth*, Vol. 1, pp. 8–41, London: Chapman & Hall.

Robinson, S. (1989b) The role of the midwife: opportunities and constraints. In Chalmers, I., Enkin, M. and Kierse, M.J.N.C. (eds) *Effective Care in Pregnancy and Childbirth*, pp. 162–80, Oxford: Oxford Medical.

Royal College of General Practitioners and Royal College of Obstetricians and Gynaecologists (1993) *General Practitioner Vocational Training in Obstetrics and Gynaecology*, London: RCGP.

Royal College of Midwives (1993) *Guidelines for the Provision of Midwifery Education*, London: RCM.

Scottish Office (1994) *Nursing and Midwifery Education in Scotland: Options for the Future*, Edinburgh: Scottish Office.

Select Committee (1992) *Second Report: Maternity Services*, London: HMSO.

Silverton, L.I. (1988) *Midwifery Education in the USA*, Swansea: School of Social Studies, University College of Swansea.

Smith, L. (1990) 'Is There a Future for General Practitioner Obstetricians?' *Association for General Practice Maternity Care Newsletter*, No. 2, August, pp. 2–3.

Smith, L. (1991) GP trainees' views on hospital obstetric vocational training, *British Medical Journal* **303**: 1447–52.

United Kingdom Central Council (1991) *Midwives Rules*, London: UKCC.

United Kingdom Central Council (1992) *Code of Professional Conduct*, London: UKCC.

United Kingdom Central Council (1994) *The Future of Professional Practice – the UKCC Standards for Education and Practice Following Registration*, London: UKCC.

Warwick, C. (1992) Reflections on the current management of midwifery education, *MIDIRS Midwifery Digest* **2(2)**: 251–4.

World Health Organization (1985) *Having a Baby in Europe*, Copenhagen: WHO.

6

The Needs of Midwives: Managing Stress and Change

Judith Schott

INTRODUCTION

This chapter, unlike others in this book, is devoted to the needs of midwives. Usually the focus of attention is firmly fixed on the work, the clients and the demands of the organization, whilst the needs of health professionals are relegated to the bottom of the list of priorities. This is not only an inconsistent attitude in an organization that exists to care, it is also short-sighted because undue stress takes its toll on midwives and because their health and well-being directly affect their ability to care for their clients.

Although the causes and effects of stress on nurses are well documented and there are now numerous popular books on stress and change management, there is little that specifically focuses on the needs of British midwives. This may be because writers and researchers are unaware of the differences between nurses and midwives and therefore fail to acknowledge the unique position of midwives as practitioners in their own right. They may also assume that because midwives deal with birth and the beginning of new lives, there is not much for them to be stressed about. Or it may be because midwives as a group have not spoken out loudly enough. Nevertheless there is ample justification for exploring the issue of stress and change management from a midwifery perspective.

ATTITUDES TO STRESS IN THE NHS

Midwifery is predominantly a female profession and despite the changes in attitude precipitated by the women's liberation movement, women are still tacitly but powerfully encouraged to care for and put the needs of others before their own (Kline 1993). Many enjoy the role of carer and this is often part of the motivation that leads people into nursing and midwifery, but the drive to put others first can make it hard for women to recognize their own needs and to feel justified in meeting them.

For many years this underlying attitude was actively re-enforced in the health service by a culture whose roots lie in the army and the convent, which demanded and expected total dedication from its staff. The training reflected these attitudes and deliberately encouraged self-sacrifice, self-denial and dedication. Many devoted their whole lives to their work to the exclusion of all else.

Although lifestyles have changed and attitudes have softened, traditions die hard and there are still echoes of these old messages. Until recently the needs of health professionals were not acknowledged or felt to be legitimate and stress was not recognized as a normal reaction to undue or accumulating pressures. In practice stress is still considered by many to be a personal failure and there is a persisting view that only inadequate or weak people need support: 'the problem is that people tend to be seen as being one side or other of the support equation. You are either a helper or you are being helped. If you are a helper, you are not supposed to ask for help yourself' (Stoter, cited by Cole 1991).

Health professionals who are upset by some of the distressing situations that they inevitably have to deal with, are considered unprofessional and over-involved. This view is reflected in a survey carried out on stress in the public sector (Health Education Authority (HEA) 1988): 'nurses are not expected to express their feelings; they are expected to be composed at all times'. Though undesirable, this denial of stress could probably just be tolerated as long as task orientation and professional detachment were hallmarks of care. This tradition encouraged health professionals to focus on individual components of care and to avoid acknowledging the client as a whole person with emotional as well as physical needs, an approach that has been described as an institutionalized defence against anxiety and stress (Menzies 1970).

STRESS, CHANGE AND MIDWIVES

However, the climate in which midwives work has altered drastically. Most no longer devote their whole lives exclusively to their profession. Many have families and need to juggle the pressures of work with the demands of children and family life. The expectations and demands of clients have increased out of all recognition and new patterns of care are being developed and changed at a rapid rate. In addition the introduction of market forces into health care has meant massive organizational change, bringing anxiety and concern about changing work patterns and, for some, anxiety about job security.

Consumer demand

The House of Commons Select Committee report on maternity services (1992) and the advent of the Patients' Charter have focused attention on the needs and demands that women have been voicing for many years. Fragmented care is no longer acceptable; instead continuity and a more holistic approach are required. Increasingly, women want to know and to develop warm human relationships with their midwives. Whilst these changes have been welcomed by many midwives, many have also found them stressful because it is no longer possible to remain detached or to hide behind a screen of so-called professionalism.

Women are no longer passive recipients who are prepared to comply without question with a pre-determined system of antenatal and intrapartum care. A growing number are becoming active partners in their own care, wanting to make decisions for themselves and needing objective and research-based information so that they can make truly informed choices. This means that midwives need to be well informed and need to be excellent communicators.

Midwives are also more likely to become involved in the emotional, moral, religious and social issues that affect their clients. Whilst this involvement can deepen the relationship between a woman and her midwife, bringing benefits and increased satisfaction, it also brings potential stresses. In particular, the expanding scope of antenatal screening and the increasing emphasis on health promotion has increased the demands on a midwife to exercise tact, sensitivity and flexibility and to be more self-aware as she supports women through a growing number of choices and dilemmas. How does a midwife present a balanced, objective view to a woman contemplating a test to detect Down's syndrome and cope with her own beliefs and feelings about these tests and the consequences of a positive result? How does one respond to a woman who demands to know why she should be tested for HIV when health professionals are not tested? How does a midwife, who cares deeply about the well-being of the unborn baby, remain genuinely understanding and supportive of a woman who persists in smoking 40 cigarettes a day throughout her pregnancy? Increasingly, midwives are required to be open to what women think, feel and want even when this challenges their personal and professional beliefs and assumptions.

Continuity of care

The demand for continuity of care has brought major changes in the way midwives organize and carry out their work. The move towards midwifery teams may be welcomed by many, but their introduction often brings problems at first. They are unlikely to run as smoothly as the pilot schemes, which were staffed by specially recruited midwives who were highly motivated to ensure success. Midwives who are used to traditional patterns of care may feel threatened by the change (Charles 1993).

The shift of care to the community

The shift of care to community settings, midwifery caseloads and the blurring of the distinction between hospital and community midwives mean that many midwives are facing the prospect of further radical changes in the way they have to work. Many, especially those who have been frustrated by having to work in an obstetrician-led environment, welcome the opportunity to offer more care to women in their own homes and enjoy the more egalitarian relationship they can create away from the hospital. They are delighted to return to more autonomous practice and to being acknowledged as practitioners in their own right.

However, some who move from hospital to community and are attached to general practitioner (GP) practices find, to their dismay, that they have exchanged one set of controls for another. Others are stressed by increased responsibility and the fact that they can no longer take refuge behind hospital policies, procedures and protocols. What happens to midwives who find the strain too much when there is no longer the option of permanent nine to five work in an antenatal clinic?

Change in the NHS

The current, unprecedented avalanche of change within the NHS brings additional pressures. In some areas, reorganization seems to be an almost constant process, with one change barely completed before the next begins. Clinical regrading, PREP, skill mix, the internal market and the move to Trust status have brought not only challenge and opportunity, but also anxiety and deep insecurity for many.

Changes in midwifery education

The recent radical changes in nursing and midwifery education also mean that midwives who have been practising for many years and whose training was practice-based may now find themselves acting as role models and mentors for students who have received a much more academic training. Reflective, research-based practice may be exciting and challenging for those used to seeking out and assessing research, but daunting and confusing to those who are short of time and unused to an academic approach.

It is quite clear that the pressures on midwives have increased and that these pressures need to be managed. It is not possible to continue to give to others if one's own needs are not met. Managing oneself is rather like managing a bank balance. If one continues to make withdrawals whilst failing to make deposits one will quickly run into trouble. Just as it is important to avoid running into debt, it is vital to keep your own internal bank balance in credit.

> . . . to be able to love, cherish and care for women throughout pregnancy, labour and the puerperium, midwives need to be cherished and cared for themselves.
>
> (Flint 1986)

Strategies for managing stress and change are no longer optional extras; they have become essential skills.

WHAT IS STRESS?

Stress suffers from the mixed blessing of being both too well known and too little understood (Selye 1980). Stress is usually assumed to be negative, but without any stress some of us would not get out of bed in the morning, and few would attempt anything new or demanding. A challenge, whether it is meeting a deadline or making a parachute jump, can be stressful, but achieving what you have set out to do often brings a sense of satisfaction and well-being.

Problems only arise when stress reaches a level that is counter-productive for the individual concerned. Each of us has our own level at which we operate effectively. Too little stress brings boredom, tiredness and apathy. Too much in a short space of time can trigger a host of unwanted responses. It is therefore useful to make a clear distinction between healthy and unhealthy stress.

Unhealthy stress has been described variously as:

> pressures on an individual that are in some way perceived as excessive, or intolerable.
>
> (Consumers Association 1984)

> a perceptual imbalance between demand and capability.
>
> (Gillespie and Gillespie 1986)

an excess of demands on an individual beyond their ability to cope.

(HEA 1988)

Some writers make a distinction between causes and effects of stress, drawing on an engineering model in which an external stress can be said to result in an internal strain. However, this may be too simple a model to apply to human beings. Some people create their own stress from within by, for example, setting themselves unobtainable goals and standards that they continually fail to meet (Payne and Firth-Cozens 1987).

THE EFFECTS OF STRESS

The surge of hormonal and chemical changes with which we respond to stress, known as the flight or fight response, provides us with a burst of energy enabling us either to stand our ground and fight or run. Whilst clearly potentially life-saving, neither fighting nor running is normally appropriate in the stressful situations we encounter in everyday life. Thus the surge of energy precipitated by a stressful situation is not used. Over time, the accumulation of undischarged tension begins to cause problems. Common responses to unhealthy stress levels are detailed in Table 6.1. Kelly (1989) lists the following additional signs of stress:

- short tempered when normally calm;
- increased coffee consumption to keep going;
- not enjoying family or social life;
- no time to exercise;
- not enjoying work;
- increased alcohol consumption;
- two or more recent car accidents;
- disagreements at work and at home.

Unhealthy stress that continues unrelieved results in what has been called burn-out, a condition in which the stressed person feels pushed beyond the point of no return. Those suffering from burn-out tend to become withdrawn, are likely to avoid patients and colleagues and to do only the minimum. They often become cynical, negative, rigid and unwilling to try new ideas or admit to any personal needs (Swaffield 1988b).

Kelly (1989) describes burn-out as 'a condition that develops when a person works too hard for too long in a high-pressure environment'. The burn-out victim is thoroughly exhausted at all levels and likely to experience:

- *emotional exhaustion*, which manifests itself in tiredness, somatic symptoms, irritability, accident proneness, depression and excessive alcohol consumption;
- *de-personalization*, in which they treat people as if they are objects;
- *low productivity*, accompanied by low self-esteem, high absenteeism and a high sickness rate.

While stress appears to be merely an individual's emotional response to a given situation, it actually precipitates measurable hormonal changes. It has significant effects on the immune system of otherwise healthy individuals (Jankovic *et al.* 1987). For example, medical students who are stressed by loneliness, and individuals who have been bereaved, show immunological disturbances (Khansari *et al.* 1990). Thus stress can make people more vulnerable to infection and long-term stress predisposes people to a range of diseases including heart disease and hypertension.

RECOGNIZING UNHEALTHY STRESS

Midwives who are good at balancing their own needs with the demands of their job often go unnoticed, because effective stress management, like effective

Table 6.1   Common responses to unhealthy stress levels

BEHAVIOURAL	PHYSICAL	EMOTIONAL
Short term	*Short term*	*Short term*
Over-indulgence in smoking, alcohol or drugs	Headache	Tiredness
	Back-ache	Anxiety
Accidents	Poor sleep	Boredom
Impulsive emotional behaviour	Indigestion	Irritability
Poor relationships at home and at work	Chest pain	Depression
	Nausea	Inability to concentrate
Poor work performance	Dizziness	Low self-esteem
Emotional withdrawal	Sweating	Apathy
	Trembling	
Long term	*Long term*	*Long term*
Marital and family breakdown	Poor general health	Insomnia
Social isolation	Heart disease	Chronic depression
	Hypertension	Chronic anxiety
	Ulcers	Neuroses
		Mental breakdown
		Suicide

Reproduced with permission from *Stress In the Public Sector* (HEA 1988).

health promotion and disease prevention, is often largely invisible. As a result, midwives have few obvious models of rational self-care and many are slow to recognize their own needs. Those who do recognize their stress may feel it is their own fault and may be unsure about how to deal with it.

The key to personal stress management is the ability to recognize signs and symptoms before they become a major problem. This is not as easy as it sounds as there is often a difference between how we *think* we are functioning and how we *are actually* functioning. The diagram of the Human Function Curve devised by Dr Peter Nixon (Figure 6.1) shows that whilst we may think we are continuing to perform well as the stresses increase, our actual performance drops off long before we notice it. Most people find it hard to acknowledge this in themselves, but recognize it easily in a colleague, friend or relative. Being able to recognize the more subtle signs of stress in oneself makes it possible to take action before the point of crisis is reached.

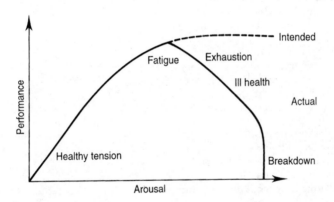

Figure 6.1   The Human Function Curve. Reproduced from Seedhouse and Cribb (eds) (1989) *Changing Ideas in Health Care*, with the kind permission of John Wiley and Sons Ltd.

Unhealthy stress is cumulative. Although people tend to mentally compartmentalize stresses at work from stresses in their personal life, it is the combination of all the stresses that affects us. Consequently it is important to consider one's life as a whole.

In the Holmes and Rahe Social Re-Adjustment Scale (Table 6.2) the authors have allocated points to various life events: the higher the score, the higher the stress. Not everybody will agree with the scoring, but it is a useful baseline. This chart helps to demonstrate the cumulative effects of stress. Events that many people weather quite well when they occur in isolation can accumulate to produce a surprisingly high score when they happen over a short space of time. It is easy to understand why a person who may be meeting the challenge of a

Table 6.2   Holmes and Rahe Social Adjustment Scale

Life events	Life change units
Death of a spouse	100
Divorce	73
Marital separation	63
Imprisonment	63
Death of a close family member	63
Personal injury or illness	53
Marriage	50
Dismissal from work	47
Marital reconciliation	45
Retirement	45
Change in health of a family member	44
Pregnancy	40
Sexual difficulties	39
Gain of a new family member	39
Business readjustment	39
Change in financial status	38
Change in number of arguments with partner	35
Major mortgage	32
Foreclosure of mortgage or loan	30
Change in responsibilities at work	29
Son or daughter leaving home	29
Trouble with the in-laws	29
Outstanding personal achievement	28
Wife begins or stops work	26
Begin or end school	26
Change in living conditions	25
Revision of personal habits	24
Trouble with boss	23
Change in work hours or conditions	20
Change in residence	20
Change in schools	20
Change in recreation	19
Change in church activities	19
Change in social activities	18
Minor mortgage or loan	17
Change in sleeping habits	16
Change in number of family reunions	15
Change in eating habits	15
Going on holiday	13
Christmas	12
Minor violation of the law	11

A score of 150–199 within a 12-month period = a mild life crisis
A score of 200–299 within a 12-month period = a moderate life crisis
A score of over 300 within a 12-month period = a severe life crisis

Reproduced from the *Journal of Psychosomatic Research*, Vol. 11, 1967, with the kind permission of Pergamon Press Ltd.

major event such as a bereavement can be thrown completely off balance by a seemingly small and insignificant event that happens shortly after.

This chart also offers an insight into the experience of pregnant women and their families and their need for understanding, support and confidence building. When you add up the life events listed in the Social Re-Adjustment Scale that are commonly experienced by expectant parents, the final score represents a major life crisis (Table 6.3). Midwives need to be managing their own stress well in order to be able to empathize with their clients and offer them appropriate encouragement and support.

Table 6.3 Having a baby

Pregnancy	40
Sexual difficulties	39
Gain of a new family member	39
Change in financial status	38
Outstanding personal achievement	28
Wife begins or stops work	26
Change in living conditions	25
Revision of personal habits	24
Change in social activities	18
Change in sleeping habits	16
Change in eating habits	15
Total	308

THE COSTS OF UNHEALTHY STRESS

Unhealthy stress takes its toll, not only on individuals but also on their ability to work effectively. 'The quality of the care we offer to our patients relies heavily on the extent to which carers themselves feel cared for. The highest levels of care are given by staff who are confident and feeling cared for themselves' (Stoter 1992).

There are also costs to the organization as a whole. Unhealthy stress is a significant factor in low morale, high sickness levels, high absenteeism, high staff turnover and wastage, inefficient and ineffective delivery of services and client damage (HEA 1988). One study found that 30–40% of all sick leave was due to stress and mental ill health, and estimated the cost of occupational stress in terms of sick leave alone at £4 billion per annum (Health and Safety Executive 1988). The real costs are likely to be significantly higher since most absences are less than 8 days and sick leave of this duration is not certified.

A *Nursing Times* survey on stress reported that nine out of 10 respondents felt stressed at work, that stress levels were highest in staff who were aged 50 years or more and that 17% of the respondents were contemplating leaving the NHS whilst others remained only because they had no alternative (Cole 1992).

Apart from the human costs of stress, a high staff turnover has significant financial implications. It has been estimated that savings as high as £6.4 million could be made by cutting nurse turnover from an annual average of 25% to 15% (Hancock 1991).

SOURCES AND CAUSES OF STRESS

The sources and causes of stress are many and varied and people differ in what they find stressful. In a report on stress in the public sector (1988) the Health Education Authority listed three sources of stress: stress arising from the nature of the work and the social context in which it takes place; stress arising from organizational and management factors; and stress arising from the varying characteristics that individuals bring to the job.

Stress arising from the nature of the work and the social context

The context in which midwives give care is changing rapidly, bringing the need for different approaches and new skills. Although midwifery is rewarding and often joyful, from time to time most midwives are faced with traumatic and stressful situations. For example, being involved in the birth of a stillborn baby or the antenatal diagnosis of a fetal anomaly incompatible with life can be devastating. Midwives who care for socially disadvantaged or homeless women are likely to feel stressed and frustrated by their powerlessness to change living conditions that are detrimental to the health and well-being of women and their babies.

Stress arising from organizational and management factors

Poor organization and ineffectual management are also sources of stress for midwives. Distant or autocratic management styles and frequent changes with little or no involvement in the change process cause anxiety, frustration and insecurity. Poor supervision and the absence of positive feedback can lead to poor motivation and low morale.

Stress arising from factors that individuals bring to the job

Midwives have a life outside their work, which can be a source of fun, recreation, pleasure and support. Yet one's personal life can also make demands and create stresses that may spill over into work. Midwives also bring their own temperaments and personalities to their work and these not only affect the way individuals react to stress, they can also play a part in generating personal stress.

Friedman and Ulmer (1985) described two broad personality types:

- Type A personalities who tend to be ambitious, competitive and hard working. They set high standards for themselves and for others, and are particularly stress prone.
- Type B personalities who are equable, calm and relaxed. They are not overly ambitious and are less at risk of stress-related problems.

Most people do not fall neatly into type A or type B but have a mixture of characteristics with a tendency towards one or other group. This tendency may be accentuated in certain situations when individuals may find that they assume more of the characteristics of one type. Those who tend towards type A behaviour may enjoy their lifestyle and find it fulfilling and satisfying. However, they are much more likely than type B personalities to push themselves beyond their limits without realizing it.

MANAGING STRESS: WHOSE JOB IS IT?

Management, staff, clients and the organization as a whole clearly benefit when the stresses that midwives experience are minimized and when there is effective support. However, there is no clear agreement about who should be responsible for seeing that this happens.

Many assume that this is a management responsibility, a phenomenon described by Charles Handy as the 'they' syndrome in which workers delegate upwards and expect 'them' to deal with the problem (Handy 1991). However, midwifery managers are also stressed and under increasing pressure to maintain a high quality service with dwindling resources. This may explain why many managers recognize and acknowledge the importance of staff needs and the negative effects of ignoring them (especially in terms of sickness and absenteeism), but fail to translate this awareness into action.

Several services, notably neonatal units, where stress levels are acknowledged to be especially high, have been at the forefront of devising ways of meeting the needs of their staff. Major disasters such as the Kings Cross fire in 1987 and the

Clapham Junction rail crash in 1988 highlighted the effects on emergency and rescue personnel of dealing with major disasters. Post-traumatic stress syndrome is now an acknowledged phenomenon and the importance of setting up support for those dealing with such crises is well recognized. In 1990, the National Association for Staff Support received a flood of enquiries as managers from designated hospitals realized the need to set up staff support as part of their preparations for the expected influx of large numbers of casualties from the Gulf War.

These and other events have legitimized the need for support in crisis situations, but the day to day cumulative stresses and strains are still generally ignored or regarded as a personal problem. Even where staff support systems exist, provision tends to be piecemeal and unsystematic (HEA 1988).

Many midwifery teams have recognized that they cannot function effectively unless most of their members are managing stress and change at least tolerably well. Some have decided that waiting around for support to appear does not work and instead have found ways of setting up support systems that meet their needs as a team. More commonly, individuals have to manage stress and change as best they can and often alone.

In practice the most effective change and stress management occur when management, teams and individual workers recognize needs and work out ways of meeting them. The issues need to be tackled by all three groups simultaneously (Stoter 1992). Individuals and teams can acknowledge undue stress and take steps to manage it, but their scope is limited if the organization as a whole ignores the problem. Managers can set up staff support systems, discourage victim blaming and encourage a supportive attitude, but without the co-operation and agreement from staff who are prepared to take personal responsibility and action, the effects will be limited.

MANAGING STRESS: A PERSONAL APPROACH

Because no single approach will meet every need, most people use a range of strategies to manage stress. Amongst those commonly used are the following.

Talking

Being able to talk freely in a safe, confidential environment is in itself healing. It allows a person to express and clarify their thoughts and ideas and begin to make sense of the turmoil within. A study of bereaved people showed that following the death of someone close to them, people who received bereavement support visited their doctor less often and experienced less anxiety than those who received no bereavement support (Relf, unpublished). All the listener has to do is listen with complete respect; there is no need to offer opinions, comparisons or solutions. The speaker, given good attention and respect, will often be able to work out their own solutions or may simply feel better for having let off steam.

Releasing feelings

The release of feelings is often confused with the pain that triggered them. On the whole, the expression of strong feelings is not acceptable in our society. Most people feel compelled to stop someone crying, comfort an anxious or frightened person with often empty reassurance and to avoid anger at all costs. As a consequence many people are reticent about releasing feelings and instead bottle them up.

Feelings that accumulate under pressure prevent clear thinking and are likely to explode at the most unsuitable times and often with the wrong people. Releasing feelings, in a safe environment, is in itself a healing process. The internal pressure is eased and the person regains the ability to think clearly and rationally (Jackins 1985).

Supporting someone who is releasing strong feelings can often trigger feelings in the listener. In order to listen well, listeners also need time to talk and to release their own pent-up feelings. Formal counselling sessions are the obvious place for talking and releasing feelings but can equally well be done in informal peer group settings (Priest and Schott 1991).

Physical exercise

There is an enormous range of physical activities that people find invigorating and use to release unwanted stress. It is important to choose something that actually releases stress rather than adds to it as some competitive sports can do.

Relaxation and meditation

Learning to relax increases self-awareness, enabling people to notice how and when they tense up. This enables people to be aware of their bodies and to minimize strain and the accumulation of unhealthy physical tension. There are many forms of relaxation and an increasing number of training courses, books and cassette tapes are available. Deep relaxation is an excellent way of releasing physical tension. Relaxation can be combined with a variety of meditation techniques so that both mind and body are refreshed.

Recreation

In addition to specific relaxation techniques, there many activities that can bring release. For example some people find that stroking a cat or dog or knitting can restore a sense of well-being and peace. Hobbies such as gardening, music or painting can bring satisfaction and a sense of achievement.

Reviewing one's lifestyle

When a person is stressed the last thing there seems time for is taking stock. However, this can be one of the most productive and beneficial steps to long-term stress reduction. Kelly (1989) suggests the following:

- making time for daily relaxation;
- taking time off when sick;
- managing time effectively;
- planning ahead;
- noticing tiredness and getting enough sleep;
- accepting what you cannot change;
- delegating;
- saying 'no' when necessary.

Kelly also stresses the importance of monitoring caffeine consumption. Whilst people use caffeine because it helps to boost energy and keep one going, it can also cause restlessness, nervousness, dizziness, irritability, agitation, depression, anxiety, palpitations, headaches and stomach upsets. It is also logical to check on alcohol and cigarette consumption and where necessary to get support to give up smoking and to stop using alcohol as means of relieving stress.

When reviewing your lifestyle it may help to consider the following, which have been described as 'rational human needs' (Jackins 1991):

- nutrition
- rest
- touch

- solitude
- order and beauty
- closeness, ideally four hugs a day
- fresh air and water
- exercise
- loving and being loved
- meaning and purpose
- communication.

Learning new skills

Acquiring a new skill raises self-esteem and reduces feelings of powerlessness that often accompany unhealthy stress. Certain skills may be helpful in reducing or eliminating sources of stress, e.g. learning to be more assertive, knowing how to delegate effectively or acquiring new knowledge or technical skills that increase effectiveness at work. Other skills may not be directly relevant to work but can provide a sense of achievement and satisfaction that will bring benefits both at work and at home. Learning a new skill takes time and effort, but can be looked upon as a long-term investment.

MANAGING STRESS: THE ROLE OF MANAGEMENT

Much has been written about the need for staff support but less attention has been given to how to provide it. Managers and any staff who take any kind of leadership role such as team leaders, departmental managers and midwife teachers can play a key part in managing stress in midwifery. The most important step managers can take is to recognize that staff are the organization's most important and valuable resource and to demonstrate that the need for support is legitimate and acceptable (The National Association For Staff Support (NASS) 1992). By fostering a culture in which staff care for themselves and for each other as well as for their clients, managers and leaders can actively share responsibility with their staff for minimizing and managing stress.

The National Association For Staff Support (1992) suggests that good staff support can be provided through existing services. These may include:

(a) *Chaplaincy services*, which have traditionally been a source of support for staff who approach them.
(b) *Occupational health services*, which offer support and counselling.
(c) *Counselling services*, though some public relations work may be needed to

encourage their use since attitudes to them may be mixed as the word 'counselling' has been included in student contracts and in disciplinary procedures (Osborne, cited by Swaffield 1988a). This may mean that counselling is viewed as punitive rather than supportive.

(d) *In-service training* and professional development courses that help midwives to feel confident and be capable of doing their job well. Managers who ensure that their staff receive appropriate training help to avoid the stress and anxiety experienced by midwives when they are left to cope with new demands for which they are unprepared.

(e) *Effective communication networks* are an essential part of managing stress. Staff who are not kept well informed about management issues and initiatives and about potential and impending change are likely to feel anxious. 'One of the sad things in the culture of the health service is that managers seem to think the way to manage is to impart the least amount of information to the fewest people' (Stoter 1988). Communication needs to be two way as managers who are not aware of how staff are feeling or of the difficulties and stresses they face, cannot respond appropriately.

(f) *'Time out' and peer support networks*, which allow staff time and space at work, to give and receive support on a regular basis and whenever a crisis precipitates the need. Where giving and receiving this type of support is accepted as normal, stress can be kept at manageable levels.

STRESS AND MIDWIFERY TEAMS

Teamwork amongst midwives is not new. Whether they were formally regarded as a team or not, community midwives and staff on labour and postnatal wards have always needed to work cooperatively. However, the formation of midwifery teams to provide continuity of care has placed a special emphasis on teams and teamwork.

A team is not just a collection of individuals, but a functioning entity with its own dynamics, strengths, weaknesses and patterns of behaviour. A team also has its own needs which must be met if it is to remain healthy. And because a team is only as healthy as the people within it, individual needs must be also be addressed. 'Groups are not only there to carry out tasks, they provide you with a series of unique opportunities to grow as a person' (Adair 1986).

A team that focuses exclusively on the work, and ignores the needs of individuals and of the team as whole, will run into problems eventually. All three areas, illustrated in Figure 6.2, need attention if the team is to thrive and to work effectively.

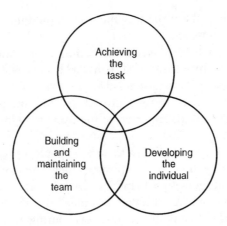

Figure 6.2 The Three Circles by John Adair, reproduced with the kind permission of Peters, Fraser and Dunlop Ltd.

SOURCES OF STRESS IN TEAMS

Working in a team can be exciting, creative and stimulating. However, it can also be challenging and stressful, especially when the team is breaking new ground in a climate of rapid change and increasing pressure. Stresses can also arise from individual personal issues and from difficulties within the team. This can happen when members do not have a common and explicit agreement about what they expect of each other and about the way they relate and work together. There may be problems with communication or with the way the work is organized. From time to time difficulties between certain individuals may arise.

It may seem easier to push difficulties under the carpet, especially when time and energy are at a premium. However, in the long run it is important to tackle and resolve them if only because the better staff feel about their work relationships the less they experience emotional exhaustion and depersonalization of patients (Nursing Times 1988).

MANAGING STRESS AS A TEAM

However well a team does its work, it is unlikely to run happily and smoothly all the time. It is therefore well worth taking a proactive approach and spending some time to work out team ground rules or a team agreement to ensure common understanding about the way the team should function and about the way members should interact.

In particular a team needs to have some common agreements about stress in order to minimize and manage it well. It has to be acceptable for team members to admit to stress and understand that the expression of feelings can be healing. Team members need to recognize that stress is infectious stuff and that supporting individuals is in the interests of the team as a whole and well worth the time and energy.

Just as individuals react differently to stress, people want different kinds of help and support from others. It is important, therefore, for team members to know what their colleagues find helpful and what adds to their stress and to respect individual preferences. This does not mean that the team has to provide all the support an individual might require, say, during a major life crisis. Nor does it mean protecting or mothering each other. What it does mean is, that whilst there will inevitably be a different focus at different times, overall there should be an equal exchange of understanding, support and encouragement.

Building and maintaining a healthy team is a sound investment not only for the team and the individuals within it, but also for the organization as a whole. Taking a proactive approach helps teams to avoid pitfalls and to minimize stresses. The following is one approach to team building and maintenance:

(a) Find a quiet, private place, if at all possible away from work, 'phones and bleeps, where the whole team can be together.
(b) Have one person leading, that is ensuring that you stick to the task and that everyone has an opportunity to contribute.
(c) Take time to get to know each other, not just as co-workers, but as individuals with other interests and skills. Take turns to say one thing about yourself that has nothing to do with work. Or tell the group something good that has happened to you recently. This is an excellent way to start any meeting.
(d) Make a list of what is going well in your team. What is good about the way you have functioned and got the job done. By starting with the positive, you are less likely to get bogged down. Then list the areas that need improvement.
(e) On the basis of what is working well, and therefore needs to be perpetuated, and what needs improving, identify the team ground rules each person would like to have. These might include commitments to:

- listen with respect to each member and accommodate differences of opinion;
- be open and honest;
- respect individual confidentiality and privacy;

- regularly review and plan as a team;
- communicate effectively;
- freely share information and skills;
- acknowledge each others strengths and skills;
- solve problems as a group;
- avoid gossip and blaming;
- develop the skills of giving honest and constructive feedback;
- deal with conflict rather than avoiding it;
- welcome and integrate new members;
- actively manage change;
- acknowledge stress in the team and work to reduce it;
- have social time together;
- identify and build on successes.

Having established agreements that everyone can accept, the group can then work out ways of putting them into action. Some commitments will be easy, whilst others may require more thought and planning. At some point it may be helpful to bring in an outside facilitator who can provide a structure for the team to review and plan and, where appropriate, provide input on ways of translating agreements into action. A facilitator can also provide an objective view, bring in ideas and approaches from outside and feed back what she or he observes.

MANAGING CHANGE

One of the major causes of stress in the health service during the 1980s and early 1990s has been rapid change in which one organizational change follows hard on the heels of another. The pace of change appears to be accelerating in society as a whole as well as in the health service, and shows no signs of abating. Whilst change brings challenge and new opportunities, it is also a major source of anxiety, insecurity and stress for managers and staff alike, so it is essential to be able to manage change effectively.

Starting with birth, which is the most dramatic transition each human being makes, people manage change throughout their lives. A change always means losing something. Even changes that are welcome mean letting go of the familiar and adjusting to something different and new. Changes that are imposed are often more difficult to manage and adjusting to them may be traumatic. If the change has major effects on a person's life, there will probably be some grieving to do.

People react differently to change, some find any change stressful and threatening, whilst others see some changes as positive and challenging. This variation may be due to experience as well as personality differences. Just as stress tolerance varies, the ability to manage change at any given point depends on the frequency and magnitude of changes being faced at the time (see Table 6.2). Adjusting to change is a process in which a person makes the transition from the familiar to the unfamiliar. This involves letting go of the status quo, entering a neutral zone and then making a new beginning. During this transition, people experience a variety of emotions often starting with shock and detachment, moving on to feeling defensive and confused and finally acknowledging and adapting to the change (Broome 1990).

Hopson *et al.* (1991) have illustrated the changes in self esteem that can be experienced during change and have identified seven stages of transition (Figure 6.3):

1. *Numbness* – experiencing varying degrees of shock and inability to function.
2. *Minimization or denial* – trivializing or ignoring the change.
3. *Self doubt or depression* – acknowledging the realities of the change and feeling powerless and out of control.
4. *Acceptance of reality/letting go* – relinquishing the past and accepting the new reality. This stage can be a bit like the second stage of labour – two steps forward and one back.

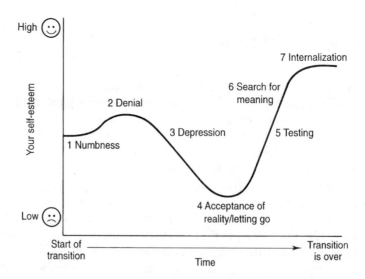

Figure 6.3 Changes in self-esteem during transitions. Reproduced from Hopson, Scally and Stafford (1991) *Transitions: The Challenge of Change*, with the kind permission of Mercury Business Books.

5. *Testing* – trying out new approaches to the new situation.
6. *Search for meaning* – working to understand what the change means and how they will be affected by it.
7. *Internalization* – the person accepts the change and incorporates it into their life.

MANAGING CHANGE: A PERSONAL APPROACH

Fluctuating feelings are part of the transition that change precipitates and it is important and healthy to acknowledge and express them. Before, during and after the change, people need and deserve a safe place to let off steam and to express their anxieties and feelings. This is probably the most important step as bottled up feelings prevent clear thinking and rational action (Jackins 1985).

If you are already managing stress well and have a range of support systems in place at work you will probably find it easier to weather transitions. However, people who are facing changes at work may find it helpful to enlist the added support of people outside the organization who are not directly affected. In addition to managing feelings, people facing change can:

- *Be proactive.* Sitting back and hoping for the best sometimes works, but it is no guarantee and resisting changes that are inevitable is likely to make life more difficult in the long run. It helps to get involved and become part of the process of change. This may be demanding but at least there is an increased chance of finding out more about what is going on and the possibility of influencing events.
- *Find out* as much as possible about what the change will be and what it might mean in practice. This means keeping an ear to the ground, asking questions, listening and being prepared to learn. Uncertainty is stressful and speculation often gets confused with facts, so it is important to distinguish between gossip, rumour and fact, both in what you hear and in what you pass on to others. This is not always easy because the final decisions may not have been taken and because the effects of a change cannot always be foreseen until it is tried out in practice.
- *Look for the benefits* as soon as you have an idea of what the change will be and what it might mean. For example, the introduction of team midwifery or individual midwife caseloads may be extremely stressful and demanding. However, the ultimate benefit to the clients in terms of the quality of care, and the personal satisfaction this brings to midwives, can completely justify the upheaval of putting the system in place.
- *Look for the stumbling blocks.* What might be difficult? What could be done

to remove or minimize the difficulties? For example, what training, information or new skills would help you to make the transition? If the changes will mean working with or alongside new people or different services, what new contacts do you need to make and what new relationships do you need to build?

- *Plan, prioritize* and, where possible, postpone any further changes, both at home and work, and avoid unnecessary additional stresses.

MANAGING CHANGE: THE ROLE OF MANAGEMENT

If change is to be managed well, managers and staff who take any kind of leadership role need to acknowledge and deal with their own attitudes and feelings, especially if the change has been imposed rather than chosen by them. If this step is omitted, it is very difficult to help others to manage their feelings about the change. When a change is proposed or imminent, managers can assist their staff by:

- *Demonstrating the benefits* that change aims to bring and how this fits in the overall aims of improving the service. Understanding the benefits of the ultimate goal can help staff to commit themselves to the change and to weather the difficulties that will occur during the transition.
- *Increasing the amount and the quality of communication* so that everyone knows what is likely to happen and when it is likely to happen. If there is uncertainty it is better to say so, since in the absence of hard facts, speculation and rumour can spread like wildfire causing unnecessary stress and resistance.
- *Increasing the amount and quality of listening.* Goodwill and cooperation can be enhanced when staff feel involved and listened to. It is especially important to listen to the views and ideas of staff at all levels, especially those who will be involved in putting new practices into action, since staff may have good ideas or be able to anticipate problems that could be managed or resolved in advance.
- *Providing opportunities for discussion and questions.* It is especially important to differentiate between information giving and consultation. Many people have been angered and antagonized when they have been led to believe that they were being asked for views that would be taken into account, only to find that decisions had already been taken.
- *Acknowledging feelings* and fostering a culture that accepts the needs of staff and offers places and time to let off steam.

- *Assisting people to identify skills and information they need* to handle the new situation and helping them assess where and when they could get these. It may be appropriate to set up specific training programmes so that staff feel equipped to meet the demands and challenges that the changes will bring.
- *Appreciating and thanking* people as often as possible.

It is important to continue these activities throughout the change and for some time afterwards. In this way teething problems can be picked up and solved quickly.

TEAM STRATEGIES FOR MANAGING CHANGE

When a team or working group is facing change, members can help each other to manage it. This works better when individuals are already proactive and dealing with their feelings well. The strategies that teams can use mirror those for managers. If both managers and teams are managing change effectively, the benefits will be multiplied. Team members can manage change by agreeing to:

- *Communicate* more than ever before. When the change is discussed, be clear about what is fact and what is speculation. At meetings, make sure everyone knows whether they are being consulted, in which case they will expect their views to be taken on board, or simply informed.
- *Listen* to each other more than ever before. Pick up on good ideas and see that they get used. Help each other both to identify the potential benefits of the change and to deal with the problems.
- *Acknowledge feelings* and difficulties. When doing this, confidentiality and privacy are vital. Help each other identify the information or skills that will be needed and work out when and where to acquire these.
- *Allow time*, whenever possible, before introducing further changes.
- *Validate and appreciate each other.* When people are feeling anxious and insecure it helps to be reminded of what is going well.
- *Identify and tackle teething problems* that arise as the change is implemented.

CONCLUSION

The focus of this chapter has been on the needs of midwives and the strategies that individuals, teams and managers can use to manage change and stress effectively. However, it provides no easy or quick solutions. Good stress and change management requires attention, time and energy and can seem like the last straw in an already overloaded system. Whilst it is tempting to ignore staff needs, in the long term it causes major problems. Managing stress and change is an investment in human beings who do their best under difficult circumstances and who form the most valuable resource that the health service possesses. Without midwives in good shape, there will not be effective care.

REFERENCES

Adair, J. (1986) *Effective Teambuilding*, London: Pan Books.

Broome, A. (1990) *Managing Change*, Essentials of Nursing Management, London: Macmillan.

Charles, J. (1993) Team midwifery: a guilty secret, *Midwives Chronicle* **106:** 146.

Cole, A. (1991) 'Pressure Point', *Nursing Times*, Vol. 87, p. 24.

Cole, A. (1992) 'High Anxiety', *Nursing Times*, Vol. 88, p. 26.

Consumers Association (1984) *Living with Stress*, Rudriger, E. (ed.), London: Hodder and Stoughon.

Cooper, C.L., Cooper, R.D. and Eaker, L.H. (1988) *Living With Stress*, Harmondsworth: Penguin.

Flint, C. (1986) *Sensitive Midwifery*, Oxford: Butterworth-Heinemann.

Friedman, M. and Ulmer, D. (1985) *Treating Type A Behaviour and Your Heart*, London: Joseph.

Gillespie, C. and Gillespie, V. (1986) 'Reading the Danger Signs', *Nursing Times*, Vol. 82, p. 24.

Hancock, C. (1991) cited by NASS (The National Association For Staff Support) *The Costs of Stress and the Costs and Benefits of Stress Management*, Woking: NASS.

Handy, C. (1991) *Waiting for the Mountain to Move*. London: Arrow Books.

Health Education Authority (1988) *Stress In the Public Sector*, London: HEA.

Health and Safety Executive (1988) *Mental Health At Work*, London: HMSO.

Hopson, B., Scally, M. and Stafford, K. (1991) *Transitions: The Challenge of Change*, London: Mercury Business Books.

House of Commons (1992) *Health Committee Maternity Services Second Report*, Vol. 1, London: HMSO.

Jackins, H. (1985) *The Human Side of Human Beings*, Seattle: Rational Island Publishers.

Jackins, H. (1991) *The Upward Trend*, Seattle: Rational Island Publishers.

Jankovic, B.D., Markovic, B.M. and Spector, N.H. (1987) *Proceedings of the New York Academy of Sciences* **496**.

Kelly, D. (1989) Stress and how to avoid professional burnout, *Midwife Health Visitor and Community Nurse* **25:** 172.

Khansari, D.N., Murgo, A.J. and Faith, R.E. (1990) Effects of stress on the immune system, *Immunology Today* **5**: 170.

Kline, N. (1993) *Women and Power*, London: BBC Books.

Menzies, I. (1970) *The Functioning of Social Systems as a Defence Against Anxiety*, London: Tavistock.

NASS (The National Association For Staff Support) (1992) *A Charter for Staff Support in Health Care Services*, Woking: NASS.

Nursing Times (1988) 'Predictors of Burn-Out' Vol. 84, p. 34.

Payne, R. and Firth-Cozens, J. (1987) *Stress In Health Professionals*, Chichester: John Wiley.

Priest, J. and Schott, J. (1991) Setting up a working partnership. In *Leading Antenatal Classes – a Practical Guide*, Oxford: Butterworth-Heinemann.

Seedhouse, D. and Cribb, A. (eds) (1989) *Changing Ideas in Health Care*, Chichester: John Wiley.

Selye, H. (1980) The stress concept today. In Kulash, I.L. and Schlesinger, L.B. (eds) *Handbook of Stress and Anxiety*, San Francisco: Jossey Bass.

Stoter, D. (1992) 'Stress: the Culture of Caring', *Nursing Times* Vol. 88, p. 12.

Swaffield, L. (1988a) 'Sharing the Load', *Nursing Times* Vol. 84, p. 24.

Swaffield, L. (1988b) 'Burn-out', *Nursing Standard* Vol. 2, p. 22.

7

Issues in Research

Marianne Mead

Research has been a subject of considerable discussion and development in the last 10–15 years. So much so that the Statutory Bodies have acknowledged this fact in the Midwives' Rules, Code of Practice and Code of Professional Conduct. This chapter aims at providing the reader with an introduction to the concept of research as a theoretical discipline. It will also encourage readers to become more critical and analytical when reading research findings so that they develop the skills that better enable them to judge when findings should be implemented in practice. It is also hoped that readers will develop a certain degree of empathy for research and the research process and that some may eventually wish to go on to develop this aspect much further, maybe even to becoming researchers of midwifery themselves.

INTRODUCTION

Midwives have been striving for some time to be recognized as accountable professional practitioners. They demonstrate accountability to the mothers and babies they care for by being able to provide the best known care. Research will provide them with a significant basis for knowledge. Some midwives will further develop this research base themselves by undertaking their own research in response to questions they have identified in the course of their practice, be this clinical, managerial or educational practice. The provision of a wider research base for the practice of midwifery will then enable midwives to be more effective in claiming that midwifery is indeed a profession rather than an occupation. The criteria that define a profession identify an individual knowledge base (Moline 1986).

In May 1986, the United Kingdom Central Council for Nursing, Midwifery and Health Visiting (UKCC) published its latest version of the Midwives' Rules. For the first time, Rule 33 – dealing with courses leading to admission to Part 10 of the register – required the student midwife to demonstrate 'an awareness of the importance of research-based practice'. In March 1991, this was revised to 'be able to use relevant literature and research to inform their practice of midwifery' (UKCC 1991).

It goes without saying that the minimum learning outcomes now identified as appropriate for student midwives also become the minimum requirement of registered practising midwives. The changes in the Midwives' Rules have taken place over a relatively short period of time and begs the question: 'if practice was not based on research, then what was it based on?'

This chapter will endeavour to provide a useful introduction to research for the midwife or student midwife who is interested in developing the initial skills of research critique. It will introduce three major types of research – not an exhaustive analysis by any means – and provide an introduction to some statistical presentation and analysis. It aims mostly at encouraging readers to become critical and analytical when reading research so that they can have a firmer justification for accepting or rejecting some aspects of research findings. They should ultimately be able to work out what is good research and what is not.

BASIS OF MIDWIFERY KNOWLEDGE

In the absence of research findings, midwives and other health care professionals have used a variety of sources upon which to base their practice: tradition, experience, authority, common sense, trial and error .... This can be easily demonstrated by a few examples of midwifery practice.

Tradition

The woman should be seen and examined every four weeks until the twenty-eighth week, then every two weeks until the thirty-sixth week and then weekly until the birth of the baby. If at any time there is a deviation from normal, visits should be more frequent.

(Hickman 1981)

Research by Hall *et al.* (1980) suggests that this model of antenatal care does not yield the anticipated results, yet 15 years after the publication of her data, the traditional pattern of antenatal care continues and, where it is challenged, midwives often question the wisdom of change.

Experience and trial and error

Experience provides useful information, but individuals tend to remember striking events rather than the ordinary and this can easily influence their judgement. The use of personal experience as a basis for knowledge is too selective because it does not usually allow the practitioner to put information into perspective. 'In hindsight, people consistently exaggerate what could have been anticipated in foresight. The very knowledge that gives us the feeling that we understand what the past was all about may prevent us from learning anything about it' (Fischhoff 1980).

The outcome of trial and error has pitfalls similar to personal experience. Furthermore the practitioner may be encouraged to draw a conclusion of the cause and effect relationship between the identified problem and its tried solution. The possibility of a coincidence rather than a cause–effect relationship is not usually tested.

Both methods lack rigour and data are usually not systematically recorded, thereby making replication difficult and verification impossible. Generalization of the conclusions drawn from experience or trial and error are therefore difficult and potentially extremely suspect.

Authority

> *We consider that the resources of modern medicine should be available to all mothers and babies, and we think that sufficient facilities should be provided to allow for 100 per cent hospital delivery. The greater safety of hospital confinement for mother and child justifies this objective.*
>
> (Peel Report 1970)

Authority is a powerful guide for practice, whether verbal or written. Authority is provided by individuals (managers, consultants) or by documents (local policies and procedures, textbooks, statutory instrument, protocols, government reports). Authorities are not infallible, yet protocols and policy documents have gained a great deal of influence, often without the backing of scientific evidence and leading to 'damaging demarcation dispute between the professional groups' (House of Commons 1992).

Common sense

Whatever the basis for practice and however peculiar it may now sound, practices are often supported by apparent common sense. For example, *hot water and soap enemas*: 'It is advisable that every woman should have her lower bowel emptied at the beginning of labour' (Myles 1971). Also, *taking the daily temperature of a mother admitted in spontaneous labour following a normal pregnancy* is often justified on the basis that it is important to have a 'baseline' for the rest of labour. Midwives and obstetricians do not, however, take their temperature every morning, in the absence of any signs and symptoms of being unwell, to establish whether or not they are well enough to go to work!

The list of such practices is endless. Very few have been the subject of systematic scientific testing. Some are so well established that it becomes difficult to even question them. Encountering a practice that is quite different from one's own, but which is taken as the accepted practice by others, can be the trigger for a research question. The example of one such difference illustrates this point. In this country, routine vaginal examinations are not performed at each antenatal visit, whereas this is routine practice in some countries of the continent. Textbooks, obstetricians and midwives defend this practice as the means of diagnosing 'threatened premature labour' (Merger *et al.* 1979), a condition that is, however, not recognized in the English-speaking midwifery or obstetric literature. A systematic testing of the usefulness of this procedure in the light of predetermined dependent variables would be useful.

RESEARCH: DEFINITION AND SCOPE

Research, unlike the other methods previously described, is an 'attempt to increase available knowledge by the discovery of new facts or relationships through systematic enquiry' (Clark and Hockey 1989). The characteristics of the scientific approach are:

(a) *Order and control.* The researcher progresses systematically through the research process or model according to a predetermined plan of action (Polit and Hungler 1987).
(b) *Empiricism.* The data that the researcher will use, the empirical evidence, comprise observations that can be objectively identified.
(c) *Generalization.* The results of the research can be applied to other populations or settings than those used by the researcher.

The purpose of research varies according to the type of knowledge sought. Research can be classified in a variety of ways that are not necessarily mutually exclusive. The following provide examples of some of the possible classifications of research studies. The list is far from being exhaustive.

Descriptive, exploratory and explanatory research

(a) Description of phenomena relating to midwifery practice, e.g. the study by Kirkham (1989) on the information provided by midwives during labour. The researcher observes, describes and sometimes even classifies the data collected.

(b) Exploration of the relationship(s) that exist(s) between identified variables. This type of research can be used to map out potential areas of interest surrounding specified topics. Midwives may, for example, wish to examine the impact of *Changing Childbirth* (Department of Health 1993) on women but may wish to identify the areas of pregnancy care over which women are particularly keen to exercise more control. An exploratory study would enable the midwife to identify such areas as the basis for further research on the relationship between midwives and mothers, targeting control as its focus. The initial exploratory study will enable the midwife to operationalize the definition of control as it is relevant to mothers.

(c) Explanation of the causal relationship(s) that exist(s) between known variables. This type of research is the most rigorous of the research methods and is often considered by many involved in basic sciences as the only true research approach. The West Berkshire perineal management trial (Sleep *et al.* 1984) and the study by Thomson (1979) on 'Why don't women breast feed?' are examples of explanatory research. The experimental design is often the chosen method of explanatory research.

Retrospective and prospective studies

This classification refers to the time sequence of the data gathering: for events that have already occurred at the time of the data collection (retrospective) or events that are still to occur (prospective). Historical studies, e.g. Midwives and Medical Men (Donnison 1988), are by definition retrospective whereas experimental studies are by necessity prospective, e.g. the study of placental grading as a test of fetal well-being (Proud 1989).

Quantitative and qualitative studies

This classification is determined by the data collected. Quantitative studies favour the use of numerical data whereas qualitative studies favour the use of in-depth descriptions of phenomena.

The extent of the knowledge relevant to midwifery is vast and it follows that the scope of research is a similarly open field. The example of breast feeding (Table 7.1) can illustrate the scope and classifications of research studies.

Midwives need to know the anatomy of the breast and understand the physiology of lactation. They also benefit from an awareness of the conditions that have been demonstrated as enhancing or inhibiting breast feeding, together with an appreciation of its potential medium- and long-term advantages and disadvantages. The research that supports this body of knowledge will range from dissecting room and laboratory experiments to field studies or in-depth analysis of the effects of one or more variables (e.g. social class, type of delivery, maternal age, parenthood preparation programmes) on the choice of infant feeding and the subsequent rate of breast feeding.

Table 7.1 Breast Feeding: knowledge relevant to Midwifery

Knowledge	Classification of potential relevant studies
Anatomy of the breast	Descriptive, basic, quantitative, prospective, non-experimental
Physiology of lactation	Exploratory, explanatory, prospective, quantitative, experimental
Factors that influence choice of infant feeding	Descriptive, exploratory, explanatory, retrospective, prospective, quantitative, qualitative, experimental, non-experimental, longitudinal, cross-sectional
Long-term effects of infant feeding on the health of infants/adults	Descriptive, exploratory, explanatory, retrospective, prospective, quantitative, qualitative, non-experimental, longitudinal

The knowledge base that is required on the subject of the breast and lactation to enable the midwife to practise amply demonstrates the scope of the knowledge and consequently the spectrum of the research that spans a continuum going from a purely quantitative end to a purely qualitative end, with any combination in between.

THE RESEARCH CONTINUUM

The research method and process will very much depend on the question(s) the research wishes to answer. Research approaches can be classified along a continuum – from purely quantitative to purely qualitative, from experimental to ethnographic, from hypothetico-deductive to inductive (Table 7.2).

Table 7.2   The research continuum

Quantitative	←		→	Qualitative
Hypothetico-deductive approach	←		→	Inductive approach
Experiment	←	Survey	→	Ethnography

In the hypothetico-deductive approach, the researcher proceeds from the theory identified in the hypothesis to the empirical data collection and its analysis. This process will enable the researcher to support or reject the initial hypothesis or theory. This approach is used in experimental research and is more likely to be used in quantitative research. The inductive approach, on the other hand, is more likely to be used when the researcher proceeds from the specific to the theory, i.e. through gathering data from an observed situation and testing various proposed explanations. The outcome of such testing will then lead to the development of a theory.

Midwives should be wary of such a simplistic approach to the classification of research approaches. It does, however, provide a framework that may guide the reader of research.

THE RESEARCH PROCESS

If research is to be defined as a systematic and scientific approach to the discovery of new knowledge, it follows that a systematic process will have to be followed. The process described here (Table 7.3) is particularly pertinent to the hypothetico-deductive approach and will be illustrated by the study on the effect of salt and Savlon in bath water as studied by Sleep (1988).

Table 7.3 illustrates the research process in the context of one particular study. Variations can be introduced but the framework remains similar for those studies that can be classified towards the quantitative end of the research continuum.

CAUSATION AND CORRELATION

Before moving on to the analysis of the major research styles, it is useful to examine briefly the concepts of causation and correlation. There is a great temptation to suggest that correlations are in fact causal relationships, i.e.

Table 7.3   Study of the effect of salt and Savlon in bath water

Identification of the research problem	Previous research demonstrated that women experienced some perineal pain Midwives encouraged the use of bath additives
Literature review	Salt is believed to soothe discomfort Antiseptic/antibacterial properties not confirmed Type, quantity, etc. unclear
Formulation of hypothesis(es) research hypothesis	Salt or Savlon concentrate would: • reduce frequency of perineal pain • improve wound healing at 10 days • provide increased pain relief
null hypothesis	Salt or Savlon additives do not have an influence on perineal pain, wound healing at 10 days or pain relief

Research design	Randomized controlled trial:
	 • 1800 subjects
	 • women with vaginal delivery
	 • selection from birth register within 24 hours of delivery
	 • informed consent
	 • random allocation to three policies:
	     Savlon concentrate
	     salt additive, 42 g
	     no additive

Pilot study	None in this study
Data collection	From notes and via questionnaires at 10 days post-partum
Data analysis	Questionnaires returned Data analysed with descriptive and inferential statistics No statistically significant difference between the three groups
Discussion of results	Null hypothesis is supported, therefore research hypothesis is rejected
Implications for further research	Importance of the bath itself in the immediate post-partum period Benefits of bath versus shower Implications for nursing practice

'cigarette smoking causes lung cancer', or 'intercourse causes pregnancy'. A cause and effect relationship would mean that all cigarette smokers would develop lung cancer and intercourse would always lead to pregnancy. That is clearly not the case. Figures show that lung cancer is particularly associated with cigarette smoking and that it is quite likely that pregnancy has usually been preceded by intercourse; however, large numbers of cigarette smokers do not develop lung cancer nor do all women become pregnant following intercourse. A cause and effect relationship implies that A is necessarily followed by B, whereas a correlation implies that B tends to be associated with A.

Research very rarely demonstrates a cause and effect relationship; it does, however, support theories of probabilities by linking several variables and demonstrating a systematic movement or correlation between them. A correlation can be positive or negative, as demonstrated by Figures 7.1 and 7.2.

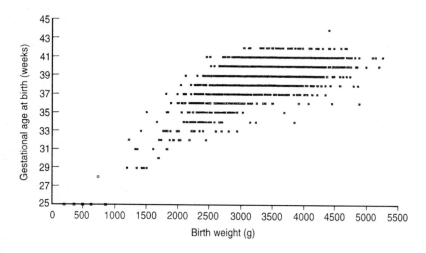

Figure 7.1   Scatter diagram of positive correlation between gestational age and birth weight.

Figure 7.1 demonstrates the positive correlation that exists between gestational age and birth weight: the lower the gestational age, the lower the birth weight; the higher the gestational age, the higher the birth weight. Figure 7.2 demonstrates a negative correlation: the more money is spent, the lower the bank balance – the bank balance is represented here by the bar chart and shows the difference between those who have spent more or less of their allocated initial £1000; an example most readers will be familiar with!

Research can disprove, but it does not prove theories, rather it supports a theory to a degree – the degree of probability.

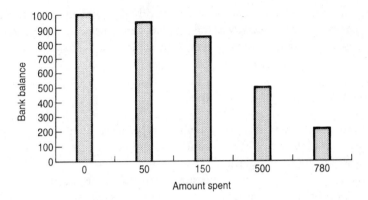

Figure 7.2   Bar chart representing negative correlation between spending and bank balance.

THREE MAJOR RESEARCH DESIGNS

To enable critical analysis of research methods, it is useful to define particular criteria. These criteria will also allow possible comparison of the strengths and weaknesses of each research method. Although we have implied that the knowledge gained through the process of research is superior to that gained via tradition, experience, authority, etc., it is essential to recognize that research designs are constrained by several factors: time, money, sampling, vested interests, etc.

From the classification of research studies, it is easy to realize that rigid definitions are rather unhelpful. However, it is useful to examine the following three major research designs: the experiment, the survey and the ethnographic style. They represent the three major methodological types. Each research design possesses particular characteristics and can be examined to determine specific strengths and weaknesses. Control, representation and validity will be particularly examined in relation to the three methodological styles under study.

Control is the attempt to eliminate the effects of extraneous variables to ensure that the changes in the dependent variable(s) are indeed due to the effect of the identified independent variable(s).

Representation indicates the degree of similarity that exists between a sample and the population from which the sample is extracted. The more representative the sample is, the more generalizable to that population the findings of the study will be.

Validity refers to the extent to which the research method used really answers the question(s) the researcher intends to answer. *Internal validity* refers to the exclusion of alternative explanations and therefore to the fact that the independent variables under study are effectively the ones affecting the dependent variables. *External validity* refers to the generalization of the results to either populations or settings (population or ecological validity).

Experiment

Classified by many scientists as the only true type of research, the experiment is a study in which all the relevant variables are identified, controlled and some manipulated by the researcher.

A variable is an entity that is measurable in the sense that it can be translated into a number or score and can take two or more values. It can refer to a simple measurement such as height, weight or age or to a concept created by the researcher, e.g. social class or high and low risk pregnancies. In this latter case, the researcher is said to operationalize the variable, i.e. to create a variable out of predetermined characteristics and criteria. An example may be the presence or absence of pregnancy where the score 0 means 'not pregnant' and the score 1 means 'pregnant'. Similarly variables can be used to indicate the number of fetuses *in utero*, i.e. a score of 1 for single pregnancies, 2 for twin pregnancies, 3 for triplets, etc. Operationalized variables can be scored in similar ways: social class 1 as score 1, social class 2 as score 2. Similar scoring facilities can be drawn for classifying people according to their income, characteristics of wound healing or type of delivery.

In an experiment, the research manipulates and controls variables. The researcher identifies several variables:

- The experimental or independent variable(s), e.g. salt or Savlon concentrate in the previously mentioned study of Sleep (1988).
- The dependent variable(s), e.g. pain perception, wound healing and pain relief.
- The extraneous variable(s), i.e. a variable that can also explain the phenomenon under study. This variable must be ruled out as a possible explanation by the use of controls (Jupp and Miller 1980).
- The confounding variable(s), i.e. a variable so closely linked to the experimental variable that it is difficult to differentiate between their effect(s) on the dependent variable. In other words, an extraneous variable could explain the phenomenon but has not been examined as its potential explanation.

The researcher tries to control systematically the potential effect of extraneous or confounding variables. Extraneous variables can be controlled by identifying the potential differences between subjects, e.g. ethnic background, parity, and by standardizing the set of subjects, for instance by only selecting Caucasian women or primigravidae. Another way of controlling the extraneous variables is to randomly allocate subjects to the different experimental or control treatments. Random allocation means that each subject has the same chance of being selected for any of the treatments.

If subjects can be randomly allocated to the experimental or control treatments to reduce the potential effect of extraneous variables, the bias produced by the experimenter or the research itself may, however, remain. Further control methods can be used to reduce this bias:

- randomized allocation. Allocation to groups is by chance only: subjects have no influence over what group they will be allocated to. The purpose of randomization is to produce groups where the distribution of extraneous variables is similar and therefore comparable. It is important that researchers should identify the outcome of randomization so that the reader can see that the various groups are in fact comparable in all variables but the experimental one(s). It can happen that by chance randomization does not achieve this aim. In this case, it may be difficult to identify clearly which variable actually led to the outcome of the manipulation.
  Researchers may introduce bias through their knowledge of who belongs to the experimental or control group:
- Double-blind randomized trial: neither subjects nor researchers are informed of which subjects belong to the experimental or control group.
- Introduction of a placebo that closely resembles the experiment.
- Cross-over double blind randomized controlled trial where subjects are allocated to two experimental groups in a random order and without the subjects or the researcher being aware of what particular treatment is given at any particular time.

The degree of the control of an experiment plays a part on internal validity: the higher the control, the higher the internal validity. Experiments tend to be rigorously controlled, e.g. pharmaceutical trials. However, where it is impossible to disguise the experimental and the control subjects, for instance in the case of amniocentesis versus chorionic villus sampling (Canadian Collaborative CVS-Amniocentesis Clinical Trial Group 1989) or the salt vs. Savlon concentrate study (Sleep 1988), the researcher must take into consideration the potential bias engendered by this awareness.

Strengths and weaknesses of experimental research

The degree of *control* is high as the researcher is able to control the extraneous factors by standardizing conditions, e.g. in laboratory experiments, double-blind randomized controlled trials. A greater degree of systematic control exerted by the researcher leads to a high level of internal validity. On the other hand the sampling procedure may not necessarily target the whole potential population but use subjects who are relatively easily available. It could be argued therefore that this may jeopardize the external validity.

Researchers conducting experiments are less likely to attach particular importance to the sampling techniques. The study group is often assumed to be representative. This potentially reduced degree of *representation* may also affect the external validity of the results.

Common sense should prevail. In the example of Sleep's research (1988) on the effect of bath additives, the criteria for entry in the study were clearly defined and the dependent variable is also clearly identified, i.e. the effect on the perineum. Even though the study was conducted in Berkshire there is no evidence that a Berkshire perineum does not resemble any other perineum anywhere else in the UK or even in the world. External validity would therefore be high. However, where experimental studies involve characteristics that are clearly not universal, generalization of findings is less likely to populations that do not share the same characteristics as the study subjects.

Researchers conducting experiments are also less likely to emphasize the description of the explanatory variables. On the other hand, the data yielded by the research are usually numerical and relatively easy to analyse. They are usually subjected to statistical analysis.

In summary, experiments are most suitable for testing causal hypotheses and/or to establish a statistical association between variables. They are strong on control and internal validity, but tend to be weaker on representation and external validity, particularly ecological validity (Sapsford and Evans 1989).

Survey

A survey is a method of gathering information on a particular population. In practice, however, it usually refers to the research studies whereby the researcher obtains the relevant information or data from a sample of the population through the administration of questions (Polit and Hungler 1987). Census, opinion polls, self-administered magazine questionnaires and telephone investigations are all various forms of surveys.

Surveys can therefore be a research design by itself where people are asked to report information on attitudes, perceptions, opinions or behaviours (Nieswiadomy 1987), e.g. Lewis' (1988) study 'Men in Midwifery' or the study by Robinson *et al.* (1983), Robinson (1991) on the role and responsibilities of the midwife or that on the preparation of midwives for practice, or be one of the methods used within another research study, such as the self-administered questionnaires used in the experimental study on salt and Savlon additives (Sleep 1988). The respondents can answer the questions themselves by completing a questionnaire or providing verbal answers that will be recorded by an interviewer. The main difference between questionnaires and interviews is therefore that questionnaires are filled in by the respondents whereas the question schedules are filled in by the interviewer on the basis of the answers of the respondents.

The purpose of a survey can be descriptive, explanatory or exploratory. Surveys are designed to obtain information about the prevalence, the distribution or the inter-relation between variables affecting a particular population. Independent and dependent variables can be identified in surveys where the researcher is trying to establish whether correlations can be demonstrated between various characteristics of the population.

In the case of surveys, contrary to experiments, the researcher does not manipulate the independent variable. In surveys, independent and dependent variables can usually be identified, with the independent variable preceding the dependent variable in chronological order. For instance, if a researcher wished to compare the career pathways of midwives according to their gender, the independent variable would be the gender itself, either male or female, but the dependent variable could be identified as clinical grade, income or years of clinical practice and its relation to grading or promotion. In this case, the gender characteristic was not manipulated by the researcher and pre-existed the entry of the individual in the midwifery profession.

Within the context of research, a population is defined as a group of subjects or settings that share one or several particular characteristics, e.g. male midwives, primigravidae, age groups, midwives working in the community or in hospital and pre-registration or post-registration student midwives. A sample is a proportion of that population which is selected to be surveyed for the purpose of obtaining information on the population as a whole. Sampling is therefore a very important consideration in surveys.

Surveys are a well-known form of data collection and are generally a popular method of data collection. This is explained by its advantages. It is a flexible approach and can reach a wide variety of audiences. Surveys can provide accurate and extensive information on populations through the use of relatively small samples. They tend to be seen as relatively economical compared with experiments. On the other hand, surveys have some major inherent disadvantages: both respondents and interviewers can introduce strong biases, and designing questions that are impartial is extremely difficult. Respondents can provide socially acceptable answers that might not necessarily reveal their own beliefs, opinions or behaviours. Interviewers may introduce biases through their formulation of the question or the intonation of their voice as well as through their personal selection of the sample. Researchers must try to ensure that these biases are minimized to increase the internal and external validity of their study.

Various designs can be selected by researchers undertaking a survey:

- *Cross-sectional design*: tests one particular sample on one occasion, e.g. the study on third day blues (Levy 1986).
- *Time series*: an equivalent sample of a population is examined at predetermined times. This type of survey enables the researcher to present a picture of changes in opinions, behaviour, etc., over a period of time by comparing results of previous, present and future data.
- *Longitudinal studies*: the same sample of a population is surveyed at predetermined intervals over a period of time to elicit information on the development of behaviours or opinions, e.g. the study by Thomson (1989) 'Why don't women breast feed?'.
- *Before and after studies*: the same sample of a population is surveyed to elicit the effect of a particular event or stimulus. This type of study can be seen as closely related to the experimental design, except that the research notes that an event has occurred but is not operational in making this event occur. Such surveys have therefore occasionally been classified as quasi-experiments.

Control is a major feature of experiments. It engenders strong internal validity, but rather weaker external validity. By contrast, control is not given such prevalence in surveys as the control of competing hypotheses is weaker. On the other hand, representation, which is a weaker feature of an experiment, is a strong characteristic of surveys. These characteristics will reduce their internal validity, but will increase their external validity, whether population or ecological validity.

Representation is achieved by accurate sampling of the population under study. In exceptional circumstances the survey is required to cover the whole population. This is the case of a Census. More commonly the researcher is able to select a sample that will represent the population under study. Sampling also needs to be efficient so that the researcher does not collect information from a wider sample than necessary. The perfect sample will therefore provide true representation of the population under study without introducing either unnecessary heterogeneity, i.e. excluding from the sample the subjects who would not add to the overall picture provided by the sample, or unwanted homogeneity (Swift 1989). Unwanted homogeneity would be found if on selecting a sample of midwives to represent the overall midwifery profession, the researcher only selected purposefully or by chance only midwives working at the Royal College of Midwives headquarters or midwives working in a remote GP unit in a rural practice in Wales or Scotland. These samples of midwives would not truly represent the whole population of practising midwives.

Sampling is therefore a major part of any survey. There are two major aspects of sampling design: the selection of the sample itself and the process by which estimates of population values are drawn from the sample (Calder 1989). There are also two major types of samples: probability and non-probability samples. In probability samples, all members of the populations have a known chance of being selected. Such sampling techniques include random selection or systematic selection. In non-probability samples, the chance of selection may be unknown or some population members be assured of being excluded or included (Calder 1989). Such sampling techniques include snowball samples, volunteer samples, case study samples or quota sampling. Sampling, however carefully done, carries the risk of not truly representing the population. Slight deviations from the actual population measurements will inevitably be present when only sample measurements are done. This will be reflected in statistical analysis, in particular in the calculation of the *standard error*.

Apart from problems of design and selection, the researcher undertaking a survey also needs to pay attention to the research schedule, i.e. the questions that will be used for the questionnaire or interview. Obviously the decision of using either questionnaire or interview must also be answered. Both methods have their advantages and disadvantages.

Questionnaires are relatively cheap to administer and do not include the presence of a third party. On the other hand, the written word may mean that a proportion of the population cannot be reached for a variety of reasons: people who do not understand the language, who are not sufficiently literate, who are blind, who are too old or too young. The researcher also relies on the probability that the respondents will understand the questions, but if they do not, they cannot ask for further explanation. Two types of answers can then follow: either no answer or an answer that may not really correspond to the question. The researcher will also have to find the right balance between the length of the questionnaire and its possible effect on the response rate. If it is too long respondents might feel threatened or not wish to give it the required time; too short and they might feel that it does not justify 'wasting' their time either.

Interviews also carry advantages and disadvantages. They are more expensive to carry out and interviewers must be trained to reduce the interviewer bias, i.e. the influence that they can bring to bear on the respondents by their posture, intonation, reaction to answers, etc.

To try to eliminate the potential errors brought in through poor interviewing technique, or questionnaire design, researchers run pilot studies. A pilot study is part of the preparatory work that will enable the researcher to select the most adequate questionnaire schedule – open or closed questions, order, structured or unstructured interview – to test the hypothesis with the introduction of as little bias as possible. This work can take a great deal of time, effort, patience and resources but is an essential feature of survey research.

Strengths and weakness of the survey design

Surveys are particularly suited to large-scale studies, to the establishment of statistical associations between variables and to the cross-validation of results obtained by other methods on large representative samples (Sapsford and Evans 1989). They tend to put a great deal of emphasis on reliability and on generalization. On the other hand, little importance is given to the setting in descriptive studies. Greater emphasis is placed on the research tool, e.g. the questionnaire or interview schedule, than on the effect of the administration of the tool on the respondents. Data tend to be numerical and therefore easily subjected to statistical description and analysis.

In summary, the strongest point of surveys is their high population validity, which is achieved through correct identification of the relevant population and adequate sampling. Ecological validity, i.e. generalization to settings, is relatively poor.

Ethnography

Ethnography is a branch of anthropology and used to mean the study of institutions or customs in small, well-defined communities. Such communities used to be small and usually culturally different from that of the researcher. British social anthropologists have claimed that Bronislaw Malinowski was the founding father of ethnography. The main difference between anthropology and ethnography is that anthropologists would visit 'primitive' societies, staying for only a short amount of time, and be mainly concerned with the collection of mementoes and explanations of rituals that they would later study and interpret. Malinowski, on the other hand, believed that reliable information could only be gathered through a prolonged stay in the particular area under study, living among the indigenous populations and learning their language rather than relying on interpreters (Atkinson 1989).

Ethnography is now more likely to be recognized as the in-depth study of small groups of people working or living within a more complex organization or society. The researcher is likely to be interested in the types and meaning of social interactions. The researcher can adopt a variety of approaches, such as observation, participation, in-depth interviews or document analysis, to collect the relevant data.

This type of research has also been called 'illuminative' and the main features of the methodology involved in illuminative evaluation are that it is practitioner-oriented, problem-centred, cross-disciplinary and heuristically organized, i.e. the research issues are progressively redefined as the study goes on and new data emerge (Herbert 1990).

The purpose of ethnographic research has essentially been descriptive. Ethnographers are concerned with description and understanding of a phenomenon through the perspective of the people being studied rather than the testing of a cause and effect theory. This type of research is therefore best identified as belonging to the qualitative, inductive end of the research continuum. This type of research is also much more likely to be conducted in the field, although not exclusively so, and the research design will be a function of the number of decisions that will have to be taken as the project evolves.

This apparent lack of conformity on the part of the researcher is matched by a set of general commitments, which can be identified as follows:

- understanding and interpreting social action;
- process;
- naturalism;
- holism;
- multiple perspectives (Atkinson 1989).

Understanding and interpreting social action.   The social world is essentially different from the natural world because it is a world of interpretation and meanings. People differ from objects in their ability to interpret their own actions and those of others, to act on their understandings and to endow their lives and action with meaning (Atkinson 1989). It can therefore be argued that the social world of a particular culture is a socially constructed one and that each person's action within that social world is inextricably linked to the meaning that person attaches to the situation. The explanation-by-understanding of a phenomenon places particular emphasis on the actor's interpretation and understanding of what is going on in any social interaction.

Davies (1990) justifies the use of ethnography as a research design when exploring student midwives' transition from competent nurses to novice midwives: 'The study showed how they actively constructed and reconstructed their alien world in the first few months of their midwifery course.'

Process.   For ethnographers, meanings and interpretations are not fixed entities, but they are generated through social interaction and may change over the course of interaction. Similarly, actors' identities are subject to processes of becoming rather than being fixed and static. This aspect of ethnographic research is well illustrated in the study of identity within a criminal abortion clinic set-up (Ball 1972).

Naturalism.   Ethnographers recognize that the actions of individuals are inextricably linked to the social context in which they live and act at the time of the study itself. Consequently they advocate the study of people in their natural milieu, with the minimum of interference or interaction so as to minimize the bias of the research process itself on the life of those studied. This practice tends to increase the external ecological validity of the research findings.

Holism.   The actions of individuals can only be explained as they relate to the culture and subculture as a whole. In other words, the actions of individuals are partly reflected by events outside themselves and cannot be understood outside this context (Atkinson 1989). A holistic view, which takes into consideration the wider condition into which the individual actors play, is therefore essential if one is to truly appreciate the behaviour or action of individuals.

Multiple perspectives.   Situations and behaviours can be understood from various points of view and these different perspectives would give different dimensions to a similar action or behaviour. To negate the effect that the perspective of the researcher would bring to the analysis of a situation, ethnographers attempt to understand and explain actions and behaviours in terms of the actors' own terms of reference. This enables them to distinguish between the explanations given by people when asked why they do what they do and the explanations arrived at through a careful analysis of the action, the actors, the situation and the social context within which the action is taking place. This aspect of ethnographic research is particularly useful when researchers aim at trying to explain 'deviant' behaviour. A behaviour can be said to be deviant in this context when there is a discrepancy between what people do and say they do.

Ethnography uses an inductive rather than deductive approach to the formulation of new knowledge. Ethnographers may run the risk of generating theories that might be biased by their own perspective and interpretation of the findings. To avoid this, they follow a rigorous and systematic approach.

First of all the researcher needs to access the field in order to gather the relevant data from the insiders. This access has been described by Gold (1958). Four main options are open to the researchers:

- complete participant;
- participant as observer;
- observer as participant;
- complete observer.

The options of complete participant or participant as observer mean that the research can be comparatively more involved and demonstrate a higher degree of subjectivity and sympathy, whereas the two latter options are more likely to be linked with a greater degree of detachment leading to more objectivity and empathy (Atkinson 1989). In the context of midwifery, it is easy to see that being a midwife may have both advantages and disadvantages for the researcher.

As in all research methods, the level of structure of observation and/or participation leads to more or less trade-offs. At the observation end of the observation–participation continuum, the researcher can select a completely unstructured method of data gathering where much of the potential information is recorded. This may lead to overload on the part of the researcher as he/she tries to take in too much information at any one time. The process of focusing will, however, partially solve this problem. The use of several observers may also deal with this potential problem.

In semi-structured observation schedules, the researcher may demonstrate excessive bias by becoming too selective at the cost of leaving out of the analysis items that might provide new light. Having several observers cross-checking their records may help deal with this potential bias.

Structured observation schedules enable the researcher to compare different settings using the same criteria. However, given the differences in situations, it is possible that the schedule might not fit all settings or that the researcher might ignore potentially useful information to keep to the schedule. Categorization may also be more problematic. These potential problems can be partly solved by having more than one observer or by using alternative supplementary data-gathering tools, such as cassette or video equipment and/or by training the observers to identify different categories.

At the other end of the continuum, the researcher becomes a participant within the study, either as complete or observing participant. In some instances, the participation is fully acknowledged; in others it may be hidden. In such cases, the subjects or actors under investigation are not aware of the study being carried out. This situation leads to ethical problems, which will be examined later.

If a researcher becomes a participant, it is possible that this participation might lead to some important events being missed. It is also possible that such participation may bias the actual behaviour of the group, i.e. the group no longer behaves as it would have done had the researcher not been present. The researcher also runs the risk of 'going native', i.e. identifying more with the group and losing the necessary degree of objectivity. This can be addressed by encouraging the researcher to debrief regularly with a colleague. On the other hand, the mere presence of an observer may make some group members feel uncomfortable, leading to a potential alteration in their behaviour. This can be addressed by familiarizing the group with the observer so that the presence of the observer is no longer seen as a potential threat to the group or to their behaviour.

Following the initial *access to the field*, which will have been rationally determined, the researcher begins to *gather data*. The research will endeavour to collect as accurate and precise data as possible, irrespective of the technique used to gather the data, be it, for example, notes collecting, cassette or video recording. From these data or from continued observation, the researcher will be able to *generate categories*. These should emerge from the data rather than from the researcher's preconceived ideas and suppositions. These categories will enable the researcher to begin to *formulate some propositions or working hypotheses* which will then have to be tested. However, this stage is not reached until considerable exploratory investigation has taken place. This stage is referred to as *progressive focusing*. At this stage the researcher is able to formulate the beginning of a theoretical framework, which can then be refined and tested further. This process is called *theoretical sampling* and has been well explained by Sapsford and Abbott (1992).

Having generated tentative working hypotheses, the researcher tests them by looking for *falsifying evidence*. Karl Popper, an Austrian born and now British philosopher, has claimed that hypotheses should be submitted to rigorous and systematic testing in an attempt to show that they are wrong; so a hypothesis must be formulated in such a way that it can be rejected. Indeed, for Popper, a theory that is not falsifiable is not scientific. Popper goes as far as to suggest that researchers should not look for confirmation of their hypotheses but for refutations (Jupp and Miller 1980).

In the ideal situation, this process of data gathering, classification, focusing, generation of hypotheses and testing of hypotheses is repeated until no further counter-explanations are encountered and all sources of likely negative evidence have been explored. In the reality of some situations, the process is often interrupted when the researcher runs out of time or financial resources.

In experimental studies and surveys, the allocation or selection of the samples were critical considerations. To enable the researcher to select an adequate sample, information regarding the total population and the organization of the field of study is essential. This is obviously available in experimental and survey design because the researcher is examining potential causal relationships. Sampling is also an important consideration in ethnographic research, but the researcher does not possess the information that was available to the researcher following an experimental or survey approach. This will only become available at the end of an ethnographic study. Sampling in ethnographic studies is therefore more tentative and flexible. Ethnographers use the technique of *theoretical sampling*, i.e. the selection of new individuals, groups or settings, in order to test the emerging hypotheses developed following the stage of categorization. Some groups or individuals can be selected for maximum differences on some variables and minimal differences on others. This process can be repeated until the researcher gets to the point of *theoretical saturation*, i.e. when new categories and properties no longer appear (Atkinson 1989). Theoretical sampling is therefore one of the means open to ethnographers to refine and continue their study. The adequate sampling of suitable individuals, times, settings and events is also crucial if researchers want to eliminate potential fortuitous biases. It will be the responsibility of the researcher to conduct a preliminary study to enable the definition of the best sampling frame in terms of access to people and events. For example, ethnographers wishing to study the pattern of midwifery care on a delivery suite would be ill advised to only study the setting on Monday mornings, between 9 and 11 am. They will require sufficient access to a variety of times when various staff are on duty and when various activities are more or less likely to take place. It might be essential to ensure contact with day and night staff, on weekdays and at the weekend. Initially sampling is done to generate potentially useful categories for data collection. Investigations will then be continued, according to a theoretical sampling, until all identified categories have been fully explored and documented (Atkinson 1989).

The potential risk of biased interpretation on the part of ethnographers is potentially high; this might lead to a substantial threat to the validity of the research. Researchers will therefore use a combination of methods that will enable them to increase the validity of the research findings. This systematic use of different methods to check the validity and reliability of the study is referred to as *triangulation*. Several methods are available and used by ethnographers: in-depth interviews and questionnaires are the most common.

Researchers can also develop alternative methods to help them check out the potential information provided by informants. It is essential that such measures are not detectable by the actors as they would then potentially alter their behaviour. However it is important that the researcher checks out the information gathered because it is possible such information might be biased by the very presence of a participant or an observer, or by the potential status of the researcher in the mind of the respondent.

Researchers wishing to undertake any type of research must gain access to the data. This is not different in ethnography. Also similar is the potential difficulty of gaining access to information that might be highly relevant to a particular branch of knowledge. Some individuals, also called gatekeepers, have more power than others in allowing or preventing access to information. It is very important that researchers become aware of the potential gatekeepers and skillful at approaching them for access to particular settings. Some situations are potentially more difficult than others and gatekeepers will want to ensure that their trust is not violated; they will want to be reassured that the researchers will protect anonymity, confidentiality and the good name of the individuals or groups. Various midwives who have undertaken ethnographic research have detailed how these potential problems were addressed (Adams 1989; Davies 1990; McHaffie 1991). It is essential that ethnographers are aware of the potential threat that emanates from the very research being undertaken and continue to negotiate access continually.

Strengths and weaknesses of ethnographic research

Ethnographic studies are particularly suited to the examination of behaviours in given settings. One of its main strengths is the emphasis on naturalism, process and holism, thereby providing a basis for greater ecological validity. Its commitment to understanding and alternative perspectives enhances its internal validity, particularly in situations where alternative explanatory hypotheses reflect the different possible interpretations of the various actors participating in the study (Evans 1989). Ethnographic research places great importance on the description of settings and events whereas its emphasis on control and representation is weaker and subject to the stage of the study. Theoretical sampling enables the researcher to exert some control through comparative methods where appropriate. The sampling of individuals, times and events increases the generalizability of the research findings. Ethical considerations include privacy, anonymity and ethical committees.

ETHICAL ISSUES AND RESEARCH

Ethics can usefully be interpreted as the moral codes or lines of conduct that are used to decide whether a particular course of action is acceptable, i.e. right, or unacceptable, i.e. wrong. Obviously, judgements of right or wrong can be made from different points of view. One can examine the act itself or the consequences of that act. Actions could then be judged from a deontological or consequentialist/utilitarian angle.

The topic of ethics would demand a whole volume in itself and midwives will find it useful to investigate the background of theories or concepts relating to ethics before making a decision about research designs, methods and approaches. Within the confines of this chapter, it might, however, be useful to retrace some of the historical events that have shaped the ethical principles attached to research. At the end of the Second World War the nations of the world discovered some of the atrocities of Nazi research. Guidelines were drawn up to protect subjects in the light of this discovery. In 1947 the Nuremberg Code was published, specifying several criteria for research, which included the following points:

- The researcher must inform subjects about the study.
- Research must be seen to be for the good of society.
- Research must be based on animal experiments if possible.
- The researcher must endeavour to protect subjects from injury.
- The researcher must be qualified to conduct research.

- The study can be interrupted by the subjects or the researcher if problems occur (Nieswiadomy 1987).

Various other ethical codes have been produced and researchers should familiarize themselves with those of particular interest to them. Readers of research should do likewise.

The purpose of ethical codes is to ensure the safety of the subjects, given that the relationship which exists between the researcher and the subjects can lead to a potential imbalance of power. It is therefore essential to ensure that subjects only participate after receiving full information regarding the study; they should also be protected from harm and if this is inevitable, compensation may be discussed. Lastly, privacy, anonymity and confidentiality should be fully respected.

It is useful to remember that several research projects have used methods that were subsequently found to be extremely doubtful in terms of their ethical integrity. Many of these were conducted in the USA; for example, the Milgram experiment on the study of obedience (1963) and various experiments on syphillis, cancer, pain or hepatitis (Nieswiadomy 1987).

The various research designs examined in this chapter each present different ethical dilemmas for the researchers. It is not our purpose to examine these in detail at this stage. However, it is essential to remember that any research involving patients as subjects or accessing clinical areas must be subjected to the scrutiny of ethical committees. These should exist in all District Health Authorities or NHS Trusts.

INTRODUCTION TO STATISTICS

In the plural form the word 'statistics' refers to numerical characteristics of samples. In the singular form, 'statistics' means a branch of mathematics that is used to summarize and present numerical data.

Statistical symbols

The word 'parameters' is used for the numerical characteristics of populations and the word 'statistics' for those of samples. This difference is reflected in the different symbols used (Table 7.4).

Classification of statistics

Descriptive statistics deals with the methods of compilation and presentation of data in order to display the most important features of the data and reduce them

Table 7.4   Statistical symbols. The Greek alphabet is used to designate population parameters, while letters from the English alphabet are used for sample parameters.

	Population symbols	*Sample symbols*
Mean	μ	X
Standard deviation	σ	s, SD
Variance	σ^2	s^2, SD^2

to manageable proportions (Hannagan 1986). These statistics can demonstrate variations in data but cannot provide the researcher or the reader with an appreciation of how statistically significant these differences are.

Analytical or inferential statistics refers to the methods used to infer properties of a population on the basis of known sample results. These methods are based on the theory of probability (Hannagan 1986) and enable researchers and readers to make judgements on the significance of the results as tested with the use of statistics.

Descriptive statistics

Descriptive statistics can be subdivided into four groups according to the summary functions they provide.

Measures to condense data

A large amount of data can be condensed into a more understandable form. In this case statistics are used to summarize and condense data through frequency distribution, frequency counts, graphic presentation and percentages. Tables 7.5 and 7.6 and Figures 7.3 to 7.6 show how information (e.g. the ethnic background of mothers in four unidentified maternity units in 1994) in a variety of different forms.

Table 7.5   Table of frequency counts

Ethnic background	Hospital 1	Hospital 2	Hospital 3	Hospital 4
Caucasian	1823	2719	2940	2806
Indo–Pakistani	560	104	183	5
African	259	9	9	12
Oriental	105	14	36	16
West Indian	86	36	18	11
Mediterranean	59	4	14	28
Other	119	23	21	9

Table 7.6   Table of percentages of ethnic background of mothers in four maternity units

	Percentage			
Ethnic background	*Hospital 1*	*Hospital 2*	*Hospital 3*	*Hospital 4*
Caucasian	60.5	93.5	91.3	97.2
Indo-Pakistani	18.6	3.6	5.7	0.2
African	8.6	0.3	0.3	0.4
Oriental	3.5	0.5	1.1	0.6
West Indian	2.9	1.2	0.6	0.4
Mediterranean	2.0	0.1	0.4	1.0
Other	4.0	0.8	0.7	0.3

Tables of frequency counts and percentages.   Absolute figures can be difficult to compare if the totals vary considerably, as is the case if one wishes to compare the outcome of pregnancy in England versus Wales, Scotland or Northern Ireland. Percentages or other calculations of proportion, such as 'per thousand' as in perinatal mortality figures allow easier comparison.

Histograms.   A histogram can be used for interval or ratio scales where the numbers used have a meaning. In the case of interval scales, zero does not actually mean zero (as in the case of temperatures where one can measure a temperature below zero), whereas in ratio scales, zero means a measurement of a value of zero (birthweight, Apgar scores). In these cases, there is continuity between the various measurements; a histogram represents this with each column touching the next one (Figure 7.3).

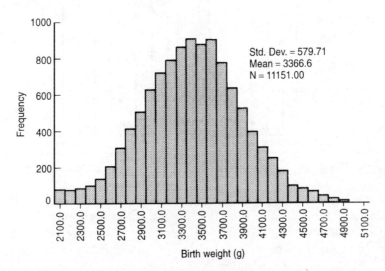

Figure 7.3   Histogram of birth weight in four maternity units (>2000g and <5200g).

Bar charts.   A bar chart can be used for nominal scales (countries, male or female) where the numbers used have no mathematical meaning, or ordinal scales (social classes I to V) where the numbers, though meaningless, can be ordered (Figures 7.4 and 7.5).

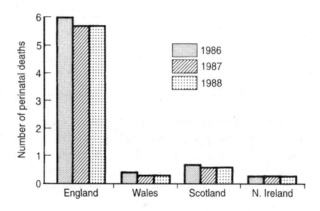

Figure 7.4   Bar chart showing absolute figures (in thousands) for perinatal deaths.

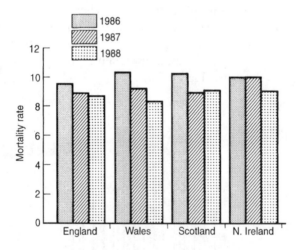

Figure 7.5   A bar chart of perinatal mortality rates (per thousand total births).

Pie charts.   A pie chart presents data as proportions of the 360° of a circle, so that 1% would be translated as 3.6°, 10% as 36°, etc. It is not possible to identify whether data is categorical or continuous at first glance so readers must be careful to examine the data and form their conclusions as to the scales used by the researcher (Figure 7.6).

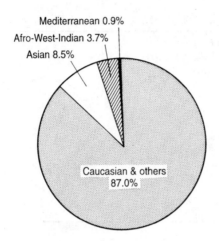

Mediterranean 0.9%
Afro-West-Indian 3.7%
Asian 8.5%

Caucasian & others
87.0%

Figure 7.6 Ethnic distribution in four maternity units.

Measures of central tendency

These statistics provide more than just condensed data; in particular they present further information regarding the centre of the data. Three such measures are identified:

- the *mode*: a score or value that occurs most frequently in a distribution of scores;
- the *median*: the exact middle score or value above and below which 50% of the scores lie;
- the *mean*: the arithmetic average of all the scores.

The following frequency represents the marks of an exam taken by a group of students. The maximum possible score is 20 out 20. Ten students took the exam and their results (in alphabetical order) are shown in Table 7.7. It is essential to rank the scores before any attempt is made at interpreting these figures. The choice is open as to whether to start from the top or the bottom score and the choice is made here to rank from higher to lower scores.

16, 15, 14, 13, 13, 13, 12, 12, 9, 6
mode, i.e. the most frequent score = 13
median, i.e. score situated at the exact halfway mark, where 50% of the score lie to one side of this score and 50% to the other = 13
mean, i.e. average or sum of all scores divided by number of scores: 16+15+14+13+13+13+12+12+9+6 = 123 and 123÷10 = 12.3.

Table 7.7   Exam scores for a group of students

Students (alphabetical order)	Scores
A	16
B	13
C	15
D	9
E	12
F	13
G	14
H	6
I	13
J	12

All three measures of central tendency have advantages and disadvantages. Of the three, the mean is the one most commonly encountered. Its main advantages are that its meaning is understood by the great majority of people; it also takes all the data into consideration. However, it can be distorted by extreme values. Neither the mode nor the median take every value into account. Extreme values can therefore be ignored and cannot distort the statistic obtained as can occur with the mean.

Measures of variability

Measures of central tendency provide information about the centre of a distribution but do not provide information about the way the frequency is dispersed around its centre. Measures of variability – also called measures of dispersion – do just that: they describe how the values are spread.

- The *range* provides information about the highest and lowest value of a distribution, e.g. a range of 9 to 16 for the students' marks in the previous example.
- The *percentile* is the point below which lies a certain percentage of the values in a frequency distribution. Cumulative frequencies are used to draw up such representation. Birth weight charts, ultrasound measurements, etc. provide us with examples relevant to midwifery and obstetric practice.
- The *standard deviation* provides information about the distribution of data around the mean. It provides an estimation of the average difference between each value in the distribution and the mean. When given with the mean, this statistic enables the researcher and the reader of research to reach an understanding about the range of the dispersion of the data around the mean.

It is important to bring in information about a normal distribution at this stage. Most measurements follow a normal distribution, i.e. with most measurements concentrated around the mean and progressively less data spread out towards the extremes (very small or very large measurements). This enables us to identify those measurements that lie within the upper and lower limits of normality.

Figure 7.7 shows the distribution of birth weight for term pregnancies. The range varies between 310g and 5500g and the mean weight is 3440g (practically the same as the median and the mode at 3430g).

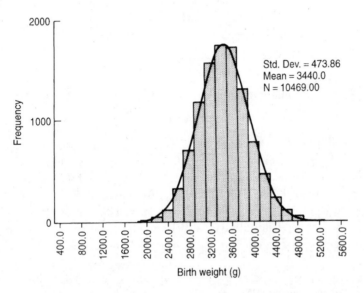

Figure 7.7 Histogram of birth weight for term pregnancies (with normal distribution curve).

Within a normal distribution, the mean, mode and median fall at the same point. This means that the most common data are also the average data and are also the point at which the whole distribution is divided in two parts: 50% of the data lying below and 50% lying above the median.

The standard deviation enables the reader of research to work out how close the whole distribution is to the mean because statisticians have worked out that the area of a normal distribution that includes the mean, plus or minus one standard deviation, covers 65% of the distribution; the area that includes the mean, plus or minus two standard deviations, covers 95% of the distribution and the area that includes the mean, plus or minus three standard deviations, covers 99.7% of the distribution (Figure 7.8).

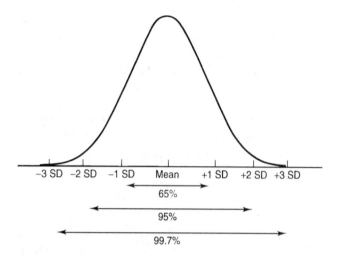

Figure 7.8   Proportion of the normal distribution covered by the mean ± 1, 2 or 3 standard deviations.

In the example given above of birth weights of babies born at term (Figure 7.7), the mean birth weight is 3440 g with a standard deviation of 473.86 g or 474 g. This can also be indicated as mean = 3440 g (SD ± 474 g). If we follow the rule mentioned above, we can calculate the range of birth weights for 65% of babies: from the mean − 1 SD to the mean + 1 SD or (3440 g − 474 g) to (3440 g + 474 g), i.e from 2966 g to 3914 g. The same rule can be applied to calculate the range of weights of 95% (mean ± 2 SD) or 99.7% (mean ± 3 SD) of babies.

The usefulness of the standard deviation can be seen when the mean birth weight of all pregnancies (Figure 7.9) is compared to that of only term pregnancies. It is anticipated that the range of birth weights will be wider since preterm and post-term pregnancies are now included. It is also expected that the average weight will be lower than the mean birth weight of term pregnancies alone.

Indeed, in this case the mean birth weight is 3367 g (SD ± 580 g) for the same four maternity units. The birth weight of 65% of babies will range from 3367 g − 580 g to 3367 g + 580 g = 2787 g to 3947 g. Compare this result to that obtained for term pregnancies only: 2966 g to 3914 g. You can repeat the calculation for 95% and 99.7% of the distribution.

The height of the curve in a normal distribution will therefore depend on how close to the mean the whole distribution is. The simple examples below will illustrate this point.

The greater the standard deviation, the more dispersed are the data, and the lower the standard deviation, the more homogeneous is the population.

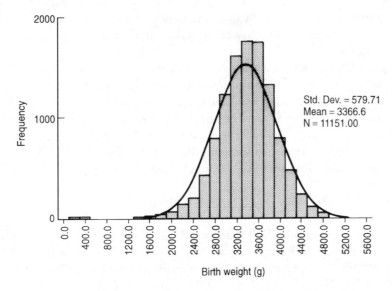

Figure 7.9 Histogram of birth weight for all pregnancies (with normal distribution curve).

It is, however, important to keep in mind the possible range of variations that are physiologically possible. In Figure 7.10, which shows the distribution of fetal scalp pH measurements, the range of possible measurements are inevitably close to the mean and the standard deviation is a very small

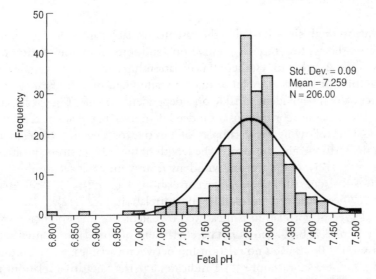

Figure 7.10 Fetal pH for all pregnancies.

number indeed (SD = ± 0.09) since the range cannot reasonably be expected to be outside the limits of a lower pH value of around 7.00 or a higher pH value of about 7.50.

Where readers of research are given the frequency distribution and make calculations for themselves, some conclusions can be drawn at a glance, as in the example of the psychology and biology exams given earlier (Table 7.7). In many instances, however, the frequency distribution is not available, but the researcher will identify the mean and the standard deviation. A simple calculation will enable the reader to estimate the spread of the overall results around the mean and therefore make results much more meaningful.

Examples

In Sample A, haemoglobin (Hb): mean = 12.3 g/l (SD = ±0.2 g/l); 65% of the sample has an Hb result ranging from 12.3 ± 1(0.2) g/l → range from 12.1 g/l to 12.5 g/l 95% of the sample has an Hb result ranging from 12.3 ± 2(0.2) g/l → range from 11.9 g/l to 12.7 g/l 99.7% of the sample has an Hb result ranging from 12.3 ± 3(0.2) g/l → range from 11.7 g/l to 12.9 g/l.

In Sample B, haemoglobin: mean = 12.3 g/l (SD = ± 1.5 g/l); 65% of the sample has an Hb result ranging from 12.3 ± 1(1.5) g/l → range from 11.8 g/l to 13.8 g/l 95% of the sample has an Hb result ranging from 12.3 ± 2(1.5) g/l → range from 10.3 g/l to 15.3g/l 99.7% of the sample has an Hb result ranging from 12.3 ± 3(1.5) g/l → range from 9.8 g/l to 17.8 g/l.

Measures of relationships

Correlation analysis.   It is often the case that variables are related in some way. Sometimes the relationship is a positive one and sometimes the relationship is a negative one. At other times, there is no relationship between the variables under consideration. It is always useful to draw a scattergram or a diagram to illustrate the effect of an independent variable on a dependent variable. These can illustrate positive and negative correlations, or indeed demonstrate the absence of any correlation. The following are examples of positive or negative correlation: the greater the birth weight, the greater the length of the baby (a strong positive correlation; Fig. 7.11); the more you withdraw from your bank account the smaller your bank balance (strong negative correlation; Fig. 7.2); and the maternal weight and gestational age at booking (no correlation; Fig. 7.12).

The degree of correlation is measured by calculating the coefficient of correlation. This is abbreviated as r. The coefficient of correlation varies between −1 and +1: $r = 0$ indicates no relationship between variables; $r = +1$ indicates a perfect positive relationship; $r = -1$ indicates a perfect negative relationship, so that $r = ± 0.5$ indicates a moderate positive/negative relationship. Various

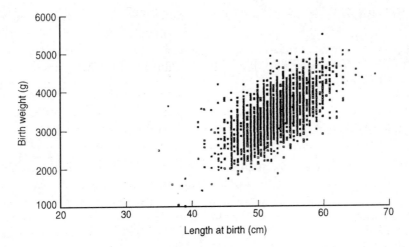

Figure 7.11 Positive correlation – birth weight and length at birth.

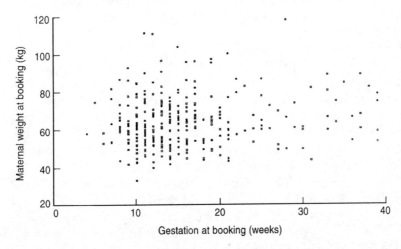

Figure 7.12 No correlation – maternal weight and gestation age at booking.

statistical methods can be used to calculate the degree of correlation between two variables. Any standard textbook of statistics will detail the steps to follow to calculate these statistical measurements.

It is very important that researchers and readers of research remind themselves that a correlation coefficient is only a measure of association. It does not imply a cause and effect relationship between two variables. Caution should also be exercised when examining the correlation coefficient of small sets of data (Hennessy 1989).

Regression analysis.   Once a relationship has been demonstrated between two variables, it becomes possible to make some prediction for future results. The more linear the correlation, the more reliable the prediction. The reader is again referred to a good statistics textbook if further knowledge is required on this particular method.

Inferential statistics

As the name indicates, inferential statistics are used to draw a conclusion about a parameter (a characteristic of a population) from the study of the sample statistic (Minium *et al.* 1993). A basic aim of statistical inference is to draw conclusions about a characteristic of a population from a sample drawn from that population. The value of the population characteristic is fixed but unknown, but the value of the same characteristic as observed in a sample will vary from sample to sample (Minium *et al.* 1993).

Inferential statistics have two broad purposes: the estimation of population parameters from sample data and the testing of hypotheses.

Estimation of population parameters

A multitude of samples could be drawn from a fixed population and none of them would exactly match the population itself. Therefore whereas the distribution of a parameter within a population is fixed, but unknown, the distribution of the same characteristic will vary from sample to sample. It becomes possible to state that a sampling distribution is a probability distribution.

Sampling therefore by definition implies a degree of error that could be random or systematic. The solution to this problem lies in the discovery of the sample values which would be found through repeated sampling. Given that repeated sampling is usually impractical, statisticians have developed a method of assessing the potential sampling error. Its calculation is very similar to that of the standard deviation calculation of descriptive statistics, as described earlier.

Although the value of the sample mean can be chosen as the value that is most likely to be the actual population mean, a confidence interval will give the range of values that, with a specified degree of probability, is thought to contain the population parameter. For example, following the estimation of the standard error of the sample mean, and given the characteristics of a normal distribution, it can be estimated, with a 95% level of confidence, that any population value will lie within the range of ± 2 standard errors from the sample mean; or with a 99% level of confidence that any population value will lie within the range of ± 3 standard errors from the sample mean.

Hypothesis testing

Although the research hypothesis is of primary importance to the researcher, this hypothesis is never actually tested statistically. Only null hypotheses (H_0) are subjected to statistical analysis.

A research hypothesis is a positive statement that identifies the potential relationship between two or more variables. The researcher anticipates that a relationship or correlation will be found and predicts the direction (positive or negative) of such a correlation. This hypothesis is then transformed into a null hypothesis which stipulates that no difference will be found between the variables. Statistical analysis aims at rejecting the null hypothesis. If this is possible, there is support for the correlation postulated by the original hypothesis and the strength of that support can be measured.

In order to decide whether to reject the null hypothesis or not, the researcher has to decide what probability (p) there is that the null hypothesis is correct or not. Traditionally a probability of 5% ($p < 0.05$) has been accepted as the cut-off point for non-rejection of the null hypothesis. This means that where the researcher can demonstrate there is a less than 5% risk that the results found were obtained through coincidence or chance, the results become 'statistically significant'. The smaller the risk of coincidence, the greater the probability that the result is very significant:

- $p < 0.05$ = risk of error is less than 5%;
- $p < 0.01$ = risk of error is less than 1%;
- $p < 0.0001$ = risk of error is less than 1 in 10,000.

Several statistical tests can be applied to determine probability. The choice of methods will depend on the type of data, i.e. nominal, ordinal, interval or ratio, as well as the size of the sample. Tests such as the t test or χ^2 represent examples of probability analysis.

CONCLUSION

This chapter has introduced the concept of research and it is hoped that the reader will already be more aware of some of the factors that should be taken into consideration when reading research. Apart from obvious questions such as the identity and qualifications of the researcher or even the origin of the funding, together with the type of publication used to transmit the new knowledge discovered by the researcher, readers of research will also recognize the importance of areas such as:

- the type of research – this will lead them to examine the research process from a theoretical and practical point of view and gradually enable them to discern the strengths and weaknesses of various methods as well their consequences for individual pieces of research;
- the research process followed by the researcher and its justification;
- the limitations identified by the researcher and the various trade-offs that have to be conceded because of constraints such as time, money and other human resources.

The section on statistics may seem daunting for many midwives and this is understandable because the topic has only recently become part of the content of a midwifery course. However, it is hoped that the approach used will be useful in introducing some statistical concepts which are as important as the various methods, since very often it is the statistical analysis that will enable researchers to draw 'statistically significant' conclusions about their studies.

Becoming a critical reader of research will enable the midwife to become a critical user of research findings and thereby increase the quality of professional judgement and accountability. This should then increase the quality of the care provided by individual midwives and hopefully, in the longer term, enable a general improvement of care through the dissemination of research findings. Midwives will no doubt recognize some of the potential difficulties that introducing change will bring with them. They might then find it useful to consult the literature dealing with leadership qualities and the introduction of change!

REFERENCES

Adams, M. (1989) A study of communications in the labour ward. In *Research and the Midwife, Conference Proceedings*, Manchester: University of Manchester.

Atkinson, P. (1989) Research design in ethnography. In *Research Methods in Education and the Social Sciences*, Milton Keynes: The Open University Press.

Ball, D.W. (1977) Self and identity in the context of deviance: the case of criminal abortion. In Wilson, M. (ed.) *Social and Educational Research in Action*, Milton Keynes: The Open University.

Calder, J. (1989) Introduction to applied sampling. In *Research Methods in Education and the Social Sciences*, Milton Keynes: The Open University Press.

Canadian Collaborative CVS-Amniocentesis Clinical Trial Group (1989) Multicentre randomised clinical trial of chorion villus sampling and amniocentesis. First report, *Lancet* Jan 7: 1–6.

Clark, J.M. and Hockey, L. (1989) *Research for Nursing: A Guide for the Enquiring Nurse*. Aylesbury: HM & M Publishers.

Davies, R. (1990) Perspective on midwifery: students' beginnings. In *Research and the Midwive, Conference Proceedings*, Manchester: University of Manchester.

Department of Health (1993) *Changing Childbirth – Part I: Report of the Expert Maternity Group* (Chair: Baroness Cumberledge), London: HMSO.

Department of Health and Social Security, Welsh Office (1970) *Standing Maternity and Midwifery Advisory Committee – Domiciliary Midwifery and Maternity Bed Needs: Report of the Sub-Committee* (Chairman: J. Peel), London: HMSO.

Donnison, J. (1988) *Midwives and Medical Men*, 2nd edn, London: Historical Publications.

Evans, J. (1989) Evaluation of research designs. In *Research Methods in Education and the Social Sciences*, Milton Keynes: The Open University Press.

Fischhoff, B. (1980) For those condemned to study the past: heuristics and biases in hindsight. In Kahneman, D., Slovic, P. and Tversky, A. (eds) *Judgment under Uncertainty: Heuristics and Biases*, Cambridge: Cambridge University Press.

Gold, R.L. (1958) Roles in sociological field observations. *Social Forces* **36:** 217–23.

Hall, M.H., Ch'ng, J.L.C. and MacGillivray, I. (1980) Is routine antenatal care worthwhile? *Lancet* Jul 12: 78–80.

Hannagan, T.J. (1986) *Mastering Statistics*, Houndmills and London: Macmillan Education Ltd.

Hennessy, L. (1989) *Quantitative Analysis*, London: Harles Letts & Cop Ltd.

Herbert, M. (1990) *Planning a Research Project. A Guide for Practitioners and Trainees in the Helping Professions*, Guildford: Cassells Educational Limited.

Hickman, M. (1981) *An Introduction to Midwifery*, Oxford and London: Blackwell Scientific.

House of Commons, Health Committee (1992) *Second Report, Maternity Services* (Chairman: N. Winterton), London: HMSO.

Jupp, P. and Miller, P. (1980) *Glossary, Research Methods in Education and the Social Sciences*, Milton Keynes: The Open University Press.

Kirkham, M. (1989) Midwives and information-giving during labour. In Robinson, S. and Thomson, A.M. (eds) *Midwives, Research and Childbirth*, Vol. 1, London: Chapman and Hall.

Levy, V. (1986) The third day blues. In Robinson, S. and Thomson, A.M. (eds) *Research and the Midwife, Conference Proceedings 1985*, London: Nursing Research Unit, King's College, London University.

Lewis, P. (1988) Men in midwifery. In Robinson, S. and Thomson, A.M. (eds) *Research and the Midwife, Conference Proceedings 1987*, London: Nursing Research Unit, King's College, London University.

McHaffie, H. (1991) *A Study of Support for Families with a Very Low Birthweight Baby*, Nursing Research Unit Report, Edinburgh: University of Edinburgh.

Merger, R. Lévy, J. and Melchior, J. (1979) *Précis d'Obstétrique*, Paris: Masson.

Milgram, S. (1963) Behavioural study of obedience, In *Journal of Abnormal and Social Psychology*, **67**: 371–8.

Minium, E.W., King, B.M. and Bear, G. (1993) *Statistical Reasoning in Psychology and Education* 3rd edn, New York: John Wiley.

Moline, J.N. (1986) Professionals and professions: a philosophical examination of an ideal. *Social Science and Medicine* **22**: 501–508.

Myles, M. (1971) *Textbook for Midwives*, 7th edn, Edinburgh and London: Churchill Livingstone.

Nieswiadomy, R.M. (1987) *Foundations of Nursing Research*, Connecticut: Appelton & Lange.

Polit, D.F. and Hungler, B.P. (1987) *Nursing Research: Principles and Methods*, 3rd edn, Philadelphia: JB Lippincott Company.

Proud, J. (1989) Placental grading as a test of fetal well-being. In Robinson, S. and Thomson, A.M. (eds) *Midwives, Research and Childbirth*, Vol. 1. London: Chapman and Hall.

Robinson, S. (1991) Preparation for practice: the educational experiences and career intentions of newly qualified midwives. In Robinson, S. and Thomson, A.M. (eds) *Midwives, Research and Childbirth*, Vol. II. London: Chapman and Hall.

Robinson, S., Golden, J. and Bradley, S. (1983) *A study of the role and responsibility of the midwife – NERY Report No 1*, London: Nursing Education Research Unit, King's College, London University.

Sapsford, J.R. and Evans, J. (1989) Evaluation of research. In *Research Methods in Education and the Social Sciences*, Milton Keynes: The Open University Press.

Sapsford, R. and Abbott, P. (1992) *Research into Practice. A Reader for Nurses and the Caring Professions*. Milton Keynes: Open University Press.

Sleep, J. (1991) Perineal care: a series of five randomized controlled trials. In Robinson, S. and Thomson, A.M. (eds) *Midwives, Research and Childbirth*, Vol. II. London: Chapman and Hall.

Sleep, J. and Grant, A. (1988) Effects of salt and Savlon bath concentrate postpartum. *Nursing Times Occasional Paper* **84**: 55–57.

Sleep, J., Grant, A., Garcia, J. Elbourne, D., Spencer, J. and Chalmers, I. (1984) West Berkshire perineal management trial. *British Medical Journal* **289(8)**: 587–590.

Sweet, B.R. (1988) *Mayes' Midwifery: A Textbook for Midwives*, 11th edn, London: Ballière Tindall.

Swift, B. (1989) Design of surveys. In *Research Methods in Education and the Social Sciences*, Milton Keynes: The Open University Press.

Thomson, A.M. (1989) Why don't women breast feed? In Robinson, S. and Thomson, A.M. (eds) *Midwives, Research and Childbirth*, Vol. 1. London: Chapman and Hall.

UKCC (1983, 1986 and 1991) *Midwives' Rules*. London: United Kingdom Central Council for Nursing, Midwifery and Health Visiting.

UKCC (1983, 1986, 1989 and 1991) *A Midwife's Code of Practice*. London: United Kingdom Central Council for Nursing, Midwifery and Health Visiting.

UKCC (1983, 1984 and 1992) *Code of Professional Conduct*. London: United Kingdom Central Council for Nursing, Midwifery and Health Visiting.

8

Professionalization Past and Present: With Women or With the Powers That Be?

Mavis Kirkham

Through most of history, and in much of the world today, midwives have been part of the social group they served. They have therefore been with the women they cared for in the context of normal life as well as in giving maternity care. In recent years this has ceased to be the case in this country. This process is probably inevitable and was certainly the declared aim of the great midwife reformers of the late nineteenth and early twentieth century. Here is an irony at the heart of midwifery: after a century of striving for professional status we find that very status and the structures of our profession separate us from the women we serve. Yet midwives exist to be 'with women'. We seek to overcome alienating and fragmented care by working towards continuity of care and the named midwife – fundamentals taken for granted by our pre-professional predecessors.

This chapter seeks to examine this irony in midwifery's development, how it has come about and its effect on us today, then attempts to look at how we can use our knowledge of our past to plan where we want to be in the future.

WHAT IS A PROFESSION?

Midwifery has clearly aimed to be a profession since the foundation of the Midwives Institute gave midwifery a leadership voice. This is laudable in terms of the Collins dictionary definition of a profession as 'an occupation requiring special training in the liberal arts or sciences especially the three learned professions, law, theology or medicine'. Social reality is more complex.

Johnson saw a profession as not a type of occupation but a way of defining and controlling an occupation. Such definitions usually sound altruistic but 'tend to incorporate the professionals' own definitions of themselves in seemingly neutral categories' (Johnson 1972, p. 26). Friedson (1970a,b), looking at medicine, saw a profession as an occupation that had successfully gained the right to control its own work and has been granted organizational autonomy. With such control clearly goes the control of entrants to the profession to enhance its market value (Parkin 1979) and exclude those from whom the profession seeks to separate itself (Parry and Parry 1976).

Professions are concerned with a unique body of knowledge to which access is limited and controlled by the professional group itself. As well as scientific knowledge, this includes the 'guilty knowledge' (Dingwall and Lewis 1983): the mystique that cannot be codified. A body of knowledge cannot be static and often we learn much from how knowledge is used. In his book *Power and the Profession of Obstetrics*, Arney (1982) uses:

... *the notion that a profession functions as a repository of 'residual knowledge' – proposals, ideas, data and so on – from which the profession can draw when politically necessary.*

The manner and timing in the use of this knowledge demonstrates the power relationships involved. With regard to issues such as birth position or acupuncture, medical accommodation was not a compromise 'since change was implemented on the obstetricians terms' (Arney 1982). Such elegant change of stance fits Saks' (1992) description as 'chameleon-like'. Larkin (1983) described it more crudely as 'occupational imperialism'.

Jamous and Peloille (1970) defined a profession as an occupation with a high indetermination/technicality ratio. Technicality (T) is the part of the work that can be codified in rules or procedures. Indetermination (I) is the knowledge and skill that cannot be contained in rules such as clinical judgement or the ability to communicate well. Thus a high I quotient in the I/T ratio identifies a profession. This ratio, however, can only be viewed in its social setting. Midwives may well feel that recent developments have made midwifery more professional, but at the same time developments such as clinical audit and quality assurance place great emphasis on measurable standards and outcomes.

For the client, professional knowledge has the added meaning of knowledge about herself to which she may not have access. In using its knowledge and controlling its work, a profession inevitably seeks to control its clients or patients. Doctors define their patients' medical condition and what can be said or done about it (Roberts 1985). Illich *et al.* (1977) see the mark of a professional as:

. . . his authority to define a person as a client, to determine that person's need and to hand the person a prescription.

Thus the professional has the power to define the reality that the client experiences. There is a frightening potential for victim blaming as professional definitions evolve. It is not therefore surprising that professions should be seen as 'disabling', as 'associations for spreading the gospel of self importance' (Titmuss 1968) or even in George Bernard Shaw's view 'conspiracies against the laity' (*The Doctor's Dilemma*).

Throughout these definitions runs the issue of control; of the entry to the work and of what is actually done. 'Demarcation strategies' (Witz 1992) are clearly of crucial importance in a field such as midwifery which is so closely enmeshed with the work of other professions, principally medicine. Freidson described medicine as 'the dominant profession' relative to which are 'subordinate professions' such as ours or 'semi-professions' (Etzioni 1969): suited to the role of 'handmaidens of a male occupation that has authority over them' (Simpson and Simpson 1969, p. 231). Whilst such analysis is rightly labelled as the 'machismo theory of professionalization' (Parkin 1979) it echoes our history.

Amidst all these differing definitions, Johnson (1972) gave a useful warning:

What must be borne in mind is that the ideology is espoused, either whole or piecemeal, by occupational groups who have not achieved and are unlikely to achieve control over their own occupations.

Perhaps professionalism has been a will o' the wisp for midwifery.

WHAT IS A MIDWIFE?

The word midwife means 'with woman'. Legally the midwife is responsible for the safe conduct of normal childbearing and the detection of abnormalities. Normal childbearing, as distinct from medical intervention, is something done by the woman. There is evidence to suggest that helplessness is damaging (Seligman 1975) and helplessness experienced by the childbearing woman adversely affects outcome (Green *et al.* 1988). It cannot be an appropriate preparation for the activity of parenthood. The midwife needs considerable knowledge to ensure safety but this knowledge needs to be experienced by the mother as a safety net rather than the ringmaster's whip. In giving support and exercising skill the midwife's role is an enabling one. This may be contrasted with the role of the obstetrician (derived from the Latin *obstare*: to stand before).

In order to take an enabling role the midwife must listen to women to find what they as individuals find supportive and enabling and then respond appropriately.

Yet if a midwife feels her first loyalty is to the woman she seeks to be 'with', then tensions are created with her professional role. As technology demands more of her attention in the presence of women, these tensions can deepen. Such tensions must have a negative effect on the care midwives give to women. It is therefore important to understand the nature and origins of these tensions. We can do this by looking at the interlinked agendas of the different groups involved in maternity care as it has developed.

THE PRE-INDUSTRIAL ERA

In pre-industrial Europe the female healer was 'widely trusted above her male counterpart' (Oakley 1976) and midwifery care was a key part of the female healing role. Midwifery skills were acquired by experience and apprenticeship, as were general medical skills at that time.

The history of midwifery has always shown 'underlying tensions about its control' (Davies 1992). The midwife was part of a closely knit community at this time but her role held contradictions. Oakley (1976) describes this era as one of 'three hierarchies . . .: Church over laity, man over woman, landlord over peasant. The existence of the woman-midwife-witch-healer challenged all three of these hierarchies.' A midwife who inspires confidence in women has a powerful skill and this power could then be seen as witchcraft. Many women suffered for this. The 1512 Act, which made the first formal arrangement for the control of midwives in England, was intended to strengthen the control of church and state and eliminate witchcraft. Midwives were required to swear before the Bishop's court to 'faithfully and diligently exercise the office' of midwife and use no 'sorcery or incantation'. They were also required to produce 'six honest matrons' who they had delivered during their period of instruction and who would testify to their skill (Donnison 1977, p. 6). Thus the first Act to license midwives emphasized their mutual dependence with the women of their community. (Interestingly, though many groups since have had a role in deciding whether midwives were fit to practise, this is the only instance of a consumer voice.)

For many centuries midwives cared for childbearing neighbours when required as part of the fabric of their domestic life. Indeed, the infrequency of their attendance at childbirth compared with the frequency of their domestic duties rendered them unlikely to transmit infection. Until the seventeenth century almost all midwives were women. Then the male midwife appeared: the barber surgeon whose practice centred around the use of surgical instruments, firstly destructive instruments and later obstetric forceps. Though men were first admitted to the lying-in room with reluctance, such instruments made a crucial difference in complicated cases. By the mid eighteenth century, the accoucheur, as he preferred to be called, outnumbered the female practitioner amongst the highly paid midwives employed by the upper class (Bourdillon 1988). Most women still used the services of the local handywoman who was spared the temptation to use instruments for speed and status as well as in emergencies.

NINETEENTH CENTURY

The early nineteenth century saw an expanding market for medical services and a context for the development of occupational specialization. This specialization separated such work from the domestic world, but the domestic world was women's world and as Witz (1992, p. 82) concludes 'The shift in the dominant location of medical services from private domestic to the public market arena sounded the death knell for women's medical practice'. In this setting women lacked access to both the organizational means to control practice and professional education.

The 1858 Medical (Registration) Act spoke 'generally of "persons" ' but 'although the Statute permitted the registration of women, the conditions imposed by the medical corporations and by the Universities prevented them from being admitted to the register'. Thus the efforts of medical men prevented women from gaining the credentials with which to enter medicine, the link between education and practice that Larson (1977) sees as the core of the professional project.

Historical studies show that professions' higher status within the occupational structure do not rest on technical skills alone, but is supported by their members' social origins in 'groups already enjoying high status and power in society' (Elliot 1972). Such status was never held by the average midwife who was poor, often illiterate and working irregularly: 'Such is not the stuff of which a successful pressure group is made' (Donnison 1977, p. 177). The Midwives Institute, however, represented 'not the whole of midwifery, but the views and interests of the elite leadership' (Heagerty 1990). Celia Davis has argued that a profession's ideology and strategy come not from a consensus amongst its members but 'The professional ideology is a leadership ideology, the strategy a leader strategy, or rather, it is the "official" view as propounded by leaders . . .' (Davis 1983).

When nineteenth-century midwives were struggling for higher training and status for midwifery and therefore for state registration, women did not have access to the resources necessary to achieve this. They could not vote for Members of Parliament (MPs) let alone vote as MPs. They therefore worked by proxy through sympathetic men. They did this with a skill highly developed in reforming Victorian ladies and not unknown in midwives today.

This struggle was fought within the hierarchical structure of Victorian society. The spheres of practice of female midwives and medical men had been hotly contested since the seventeenth century and 'medical men were intimately concerned with defining and controlling the inter-occupational boundaries between medical and midwifery practice' (Witz 1992, p. 104). There were three ways in which different interests approached this struggle:

(a) To secure highly skilled midwives who would have a position similar to that of medical men. The women's organizations that took this position were seen as too challenging to win many allies.

(b) To dissolve the independent midwifery role into that of an obstetric or monthly nurse 'who, under the charge and supervision of a medical man, carries out that portion of attendance which is more suitable to a mere woman, the changing of sheets and attending to the patient, and attentions of that kind' (HMSO 1892, p. 133). This option was much supported by GPs and prevailed in the USA where the more democratic structure of medicine was dominated by GPs and achieved the almost complete extinction of midwifery.

(c) To preserve the role of the midwife as an independent practitioner within the strictly defined sphere of normal childbearing. Such a role would save doctors being called out, or called out with little chance of remuneration, thus relieving them of 'tiresome and unremunerative work' (HMSO 1892, p. 22). This fitted the world view of many of the aristocrats of British medicine who saw midwifery as 'an occupation degrading to a gentleman' (Smith 1979, p. 23). There were also humanitarian motives, as Dr Aveling stated:

If it were possible, I would have every woman attended by a duty qualified medical man, but as this cannot be, public safety and humanity demand legislative action to enable poor women to know whether those who call themselves midwives are safely competent.

(*Nursing Notes* 1891, p. 8)

This third view, which was to prevail in 1902, assured both the continuance of midwifery and its control by medical men. In this situation the boundaries between midwifery and medicine had to be clearly set. 'What you want to educate midwives for is for them to know their own ignorance. That is really the one great object in educating midwives' (HMSO 1892, p. 101). Midwifery education was to be 'kept necessarily and designedly limited' (HMSO 1892, p. 121). Witz (1992, p. 112) described this as 'a demarcationary strategy of deskilling' by medical men who constructed the occupational boundaries between midwifery and medicine and thus defined midwifery. At the same time:

> *The de-skilling strategy aimed to preserve midwifery as a distinct female occupational role in the medical division of labour, permitting the midwife independence in the daily provision of midwifery services and legitimating an independent practitioner–client relationship between a woman and her client.*
>
> (Witz 1992, p. 113)

The ladies of the Midwives Institute thus preserved for midwives a degree of autonomy in the practice of midwifery by compliance with a limited, medically defined, sphere of practice. They achieved this aim with the support of sympathetic members of the upper classes and those leading doctors who would support them. Such supporters were able to defeat the opposition of the socially inferior GPs. With such support the price midwives paid for state registration was a large degree of medical control and 'the unenviable distinction of being the only profession controlled by a body on which its members must never be more than a minority' (Donnison 1977, p. 179).

The attainment of a legal system of registration was bound to have a profound effect on midwifery. Weitz and Sullivan (1985) observed a 'cooptation' of midwives into a medical model of care in Arizona after the introduction of an active licensing system for lay midwives. Such a process has been observed in several settings very different from those that put such pressures on Victorian midwives (Sullivan and Weitz 1989).

THE MIDWIFERY ELITE: LADIES AND WOMEN

At a time when 'in the context of late nineteenth-century medical care delivery, lay midwives offered at least as safe a service to parturient women as physicians' (Heagerty 1990, p. 7), the campaigners for midwifery's future were a very different group. The Midwives Institute's early members trained in the most prestigious midwifery courses in this country but few of them continued in clinical practice after qualification. They immediately moved to the highest positions of management in maternity and philanthropic institutions as befitted their position in society.

Rosalind Paget, probably the best known of this elite, came from a wealthy Liverpool family whose fortune came from shipbuilding. She was the niece of

William Rathbone the philanthropist, nursing innovator and MP. Her wealth supported the Institute for many years. She founded *Nursing Notes* and with Emma Brierly edited it for decades, and from 1896 she devoted all her time to the Institute's cause.

The midwife members of the Institute's Council were all trained nurses. Rosalind Paget (1901) wrote 'Being a nurse myself, I naturally in no way under rate, in fact I am inclined to over rate, the importance of a midwife being a good nurse'. Nursing training, in this era, strictly instilled deference to male medical authority:

Every medical man has a right to look for loyalty, a steady upholding of his authority to the patient . . . and the remembrance of the nurse that she is there to do what she is told, and not either to give, or try to carry out her own opinions.
(*Nursing Notes* November 1900, p. 156)

A doctrine of service and self-sacrifice was the ideal that defined relationships with patients and doctors. The leadership believed midwifery to be 'the inferior branch of the healing profession' and medicine to be midwifery's 'natural leader and superior' (*Nursing Notes* April 1915, p. 182).

At a time when even privileged women suffered from social and political inequality, the Institute offered a haven where they could gain mutual support and work for a high ideal. The ideal went beyond making mandatory the registration, licensing and training of midwives. They sought to improve the quality of midwifery attendance for the working class and at the same time to reform working-class habits and values. The midwife must aim 'to exert a wholesome influence over her patients . . . to raise and refine their feelings and make them see the benefit of cleanliness and order . . .' (*Nursing Notes* March 1890). They worked for this with true missionary zeal. Alice Gregory, daughter of the Dean of St Pauls, wrote *The Midwife: Her Book* (1923) in which she described:

A great battlefield . . . on one side . . . the devil sending out his emmisaries, superstition, dirt, germs that bring disease . . . . And on the other side, the Kingdom of God, coming, irresistibly coming . . .

The 1902 Act was the result of this zeal plus wider political concern over working-class health and the future of the British Empire. The Midwives Act was the first of a series of Acts increasing state involvement in public health, especially maternal and infant health. However, the missionary zeal of the midwifery elite reflected the values of its members whose viewpoint was inevitably from above and not tempered by actual contact with childbearing women. They were less concerned with state intervention than with 'mental and moral qualities' (*Nursing Notes* Sept 1903). The professional elite sought

formal training for midwives partly to change the tone of midwifery by changing its social class structure:

> *Because of their greater technical expertise and their higher moral sense as middle-*
> *class women, middle-class trained midwives could combine the benefits of safer mid-*
> *wifery practice with qualified instruction in the behaviour the Institute believed most*
> *fitting for working-class women and their families.*
>
> (Heagerty, 1990, p. 1)

In this sense the 1902 Act was only a partial victory as it allowed lay midwives to register and continue to practise as 'bona fide' midwives. This did not
fit the hierarchical social view of the elite who sought to improve the lot of
working-class women by intervention from above. It is ironic that, at this time,
many bona fide midwives must have agreed with the Rotherham midwife
Granny Redman who dismissed the 'new fangled certified midwives' on the
grounds that they 'didn't know much, how could they with only three months
training' (Chamberlain 1981).

The Institute supported women's suffrage and those who criticized the
miliant suffragettes' activities were accused of 'narrow professionalism which
never yet produced the best worker' (*Nursing Notes* May 1912, p. 118). Yet
whilst the leadership supported female suffrage as a move towards equality of
opportunity for middle-class women, 'for the working-class woman they advocated a life entirely restricted to those functions from which middle-class
women sought to be free' (Heagerty 1990, p. 47).

Meanwhile most practising midwives belonged to the working class, as did
the women in their care. Many bona fide midwives continued to practise and
the key argument against them – that their practice put childbearing women at
increased risk of infection – was not substantiated. One Inspector of Midwives
surveyed her 1907–1918 statistics and found 'The figures show the lowest death
rate amongst mothers attended by the very women that the Midwives Act 1902
was passed to do away with' (*Nursing Notes* March 1931). Nevertheless, the
Central Midwives Board and Local Supervising Authorities showed little
understanding of the realities of these midwives' lives. Routine supervision of
midwives was carried out by a midwifery inspector who was not required to be
a midwife and many Local Supervising Authorities preferred 'a lady' who
would be accustomed to supervising subordinates. This led to much misunder-
standing, particularly with young ladies inspecting very experienced midwives.

> . . . *the midwife herself was expected to conform to the moral and cultural standards*
> *of middle-class social reformers, rather than those of the working-class community in*
> *which most midwives had their roots. From this framework of stipulations and*
> *restrictions would emerge the ideal midwife: one who no longer placed the women*

she attended before her submission to the medical profession and her deference to her social betters.

(Heagerty 1990, p. 82)

This was particularly tragic where a midwife's 'offence' was caused simply by her poverty or her respect for the poverty of those in her care. Such women's lives were 'unimaginable to those who are born in the more fortunate classes of society' (Llewelyn Davies 1977). Rank and file midwives supported, and were supported by, the women of their community, as shown in the petitions in support of many midwives subject to disciplinary processes. From the other side of an unbridgeable social divide, midwifery reformers continued to place responsibility for the country's high infant and maternal mortality with 'ignorant working-class mothers and untrained midwives'. Yet bona fide midwives continued to support mothers not just during labour but by helping them with domestic work after the delivery. Qualified midwives were not willing to perform these menial but vital tasks. So, in Kate Isherwood's (1992) view, 'as well as being more expensive, they were of less use to women'. In contrast, an unqualified handywoman was described to Leap and Hunter (1993, p. 36), 'She wasn't like a paid person in any official capacity. It was just word of mouth and kindness'. This demonstrates the tension between the professional and the women's view of maternity care. The professional definition was 'official' and based on clinical need; for women their needs were also socially defined.

By 1910 many local groups of rank and file midwives had been formed and in that year many of them joined together into the British Union of Midwives and the National Midwives Association. The British Union of Midwives aimed to organize midwives into 'a trades union, a democratic body' (*Nursing Notes* November 1911). When *Nursing Notes* criticized the British Union for thus 'undermining the dignity of midwifery' a correspondent replied:

Why should a midwife be expected to uphold the 'dignity of her calling' on the miserable pittance she is often obliged to take in payment for her services . . . . Let us combine and insist upon receiving good pay for good service and thus shall we 'uphold the dignity of our calling'.

(*Nursing Notes* November 1910)

The midwife's poverty sprang from the poverty of those she cared for and the Union saw the answer as lying-in state aid:

If poor women whom we attend are unable to pay it should be forthcoming from another source . . . is not the midwife doing important public work and ought she not to be paid for it?

(*Nursing Notes* November 1910)

The President of the Union declared in its paper *The Midwives Record* 'What midwives really wanted was state aid and they must fight for it' (February 26 1910). Unlike the Midwives Institute the British Union sought to help directly rather than reform childbearing women. Like the women in their care:

Serious minded midwives, intent on the practice of a great science and on the eleva-
tion of their profession, do not need to be fussed over and patronised. They are tired
of 'charity mongers'; they are sick of being 'bossed'.

(*Midwives Record* May 1910)

Whilst the Union sought a salary for midwives the Institute responded to the economic pressures on midwives by staying true to the *laissez faire* economic beliefs of their class. In the Institute's view 'wholesome competition between midwives tends to keep up efficiency', 'independence is maintained' and by this example of independence 'pauperism is discouraged' (*Nursing Notes* May 1918). Whilst opinion was turning towards a salaried service, the Institute insisted that the mother pay for the midwife's services. 'The money is there', Rosalind Paget told her readers (*Nursing Notes* May 1918) and advised midwives to insist on payment in advance. Mrs Layton, a bona fide midwife petitioning parliament for maternity benefit to be included in the first National Insurance Bill struck a more realistic note:

If a woman had a good husband, he gave her all he could from his wages, and the
woman had to do the rest, going short herself, for the man had to be kept going for
the work's sake, and it would break her heart to starve her children.

(Llewelyn Davies 1977)

It is perhaps significant that Mrs Layton put her considerable political talents to the service of women through the working-class Women's Cooperative Guild, where she had developed those talents, rather than working to advance the profession.

In the interwar years maternal morality rose although female mortality generally declined. Janet Mary Campbell was Senior Medical Officer to the Maternity and Child Health section of the Ministry of Health at this time. It is of note that it was a woman, qualified as a doctor in 1901, who wrote the crucial reports on this issue until she was forced by the 'marriage bar' to resign from her post in 1934. For Campbell the main issues were preventing the spread of infection and preventative maternity care. Like the Midwives Institute she saw the broader factors leading to maternal morbidity as a matter of personal not social responsibility. Campbell sought maternity services that would educate women of 'the dangers they invite and the risks they run through neglect of themselves' (Campbell 1924). This emphasis on education ignored the fact that for many women this 'neglect' was 'chosen' in the face of grinding poverty and family responsibilities.

The expanded antenatal care envisaged by Campbell put increasing demands on the midwife and her emphasis on the prevention of infection led to the recommendation that for midwives to also be nurses would 'be good for the profession as a whole and the community at large' (Ministry of Health 1929). It is another social irony that this woman doctor, concerned with preventative care and highly critical of unnecessary medical intervention in birth, should produce the 1924 Campbell Report which was to prove a key early step in developing a policy of institutional confinement. Similarly, by stating that a physician should conduct the initial examination of a pregnant woman, Campbell suggested a crucial change in who defined normality and thereby the midwife's field of work.

ORGANIZATIONS, INSTITUTIONS AND THEIR EFFECTS ON THOSE WITHIN THEM

Interprofessional tensions

The expansion of antenatal care highlighted a dilemma. The law and their own professional interest supported midwives in claiming antenatal as well as subsequent care as their field. Antenatal examinations, especially the initial one, are concerned with differentiating between normal and abnormal and planning care accordingly. This could be seen as diagnosis or as a simpler skill. The Insitute never suggested that the midwife could diagnose but supported her in determining which cases fell within her field of practice and which should be referred to a doctor. Within the social and political setting of maternity care this debate has continued through the century.

The call for increased education of midwives in midwifery and nursing led again to the call to bring 'the right type of midwife' into the profession:

> *If the midwife is to fulfil her functions and worthily uphold the traditions of medical science . . . she must be fitted for her calling, not only by training and experience, but also by her breeding and general education.*
>
> (*Nursing Notes* July 1925)

Within this discussion the call for working midwives, as distinct from midwifery's leaders, to be trained nurses was a call to bring into midwifery a professional tradition very different from that familiar to most practising midwives. Whilst the authority and independence of the midwife was by this time difficult to maintain, it stood in stark contrast to nursing, which existed within a medical hierarchy strictly enforced by training and hospital discipline. The nurse '. . . is used to calling her superior "Sir" ', whilst a midwife who was not a nurse tended to have 'more difficulty in acquiring the calm professional manner of the trained nurse . . . however good a midwife might be at her work, it is a pity when she fails in the right tone and attitude towards the doctor – that of a subordinate' (*Nursing Notes* October 1931). The debate raged. In Heagerty's analysis:

> *The established relationship between the doctor and the nurse stood in counterpoint to the tension between doctors and midwives over midwives' expanded responsibilities. Whilst nursing training legitimised midwifery's assumption of expanded responsibilities, it also reinforced the medical profession's dominance in maternity care.*
>
> (Heagerty 1990, p. 197)

A salaried service or free enterprise

As subsidized midwifery services began to grow in some areas, independent midwives often found themselves in financial difficulties. Nevertheless, the Institute continued to oppose a salaried service which its leaders saw as 'charity on the part of the provident for the benefit of the improvident' and continued to support 'economic independence' (*Nursing Notes* May 1920). As time passed, the private practice of midwifery was increasingly marginalized by subsidized maternity care. Independent midwives without private financial means often found themselves 'shabby and in debt' (*Nursing Notes* November 1920). Debate raged within midwifery and within the Institute. One, predictable, reaction of the leadership was to blame the 'oversupply' of working-class midwives who were often mothers and only able to work part-time. Dire warnings were given as to 'the growth of a pin money class of midwife whose existence is a menace to midwifery considered as a profession' (*Nursing Notes* April 1932). The answer was a longer training, which would attract a 'higher type' into midwifery.

After fierce debate, the Institute leadership and its supporters came to accept, and eventually to lobby for, a salaried domiciliary midwifery service subsidized by the government. It is important to note, however, that the midwives professional body came relatively late to support this cause, which ample evidence had long shown to benefit childbearing women. By 1936 salaried or subsidized midwives constituted half those practising. Though their patients were often 'overburdened, undernourished, living in insanitary conditions and far from specialist aid' many had maternal death rates half or less of the national average (Hansard 1936 quoted by Donnison 1977, p. 189).

The 1936 Midwives Act was 'a landmark in the professional development of midwives' (Donnison 1977, p. 191) in several ways. It required local authorities to provide a salaried whole-time midwifery service, adequate to local need, free or at reduced cost. It also provided for the local authority midwife to be engaged as a maternity nurse in cases where the GP was in charge of the delivery, thus banning the unqualified handywoman from attending in any capacity. The Act facilitated the extension of the midwife's work into antenatal care and accelerated the provision of analgesia in domiciliary midwifery. In the situation thus created it was possible for the Central Midwives Board to extend midwifery training and require practising midwives to attend refresher courses.

Institutionalization: the normal in an abnormal setting

Another key issue for the professions involved around birth in this century has been the institutionalization of birth. Here again many factors and interests were at play of which the evidence concerning the well-being of mothers and babies was only a minor issue. As the statistician Marjorie Tew observed of a slightly earlier period:

> . . . *though the natural process of childbirth resulted in many casualties, the evidence was consistently that the obstetric interventions then available resulted in even more. But this evidence was apparently disbelieved or its significance rejected as repugnant to theoretical reasoning when further developments of the maternity services were organised.*
>
> (Tew 1986)

The fruits of such 'theoretical reasoning' and the victory of the medical model of childbirth are reflected in the official recommendations and statistics for place of birth.

The policy of institutional confinement was developed by the Ministry of Health following the 1924 Campbell Report. The proportion of women who delivered in institutions increased from 15% of live births in England and Wales in 1927 to 64% in 1958. In 1959 the Cranbrook Committee recommended provision for 70% institutional confinement and this was achieved in 1965. In 1970 the Peel Committee, with no statistical backing (Tew 1978), recommended 100% hospital confinement, which was very nearly achieved within a decade. From 1946 there was also a move into larger hospitals with the closure of private maternity homes and GP units, again with no justification in terms of maternal or infant well-being.

The vast majority of women in this country today therefore experience labour as hospital inpatients. Often this is their first experience of hospitalization. It is preceded by a period of socialization into the patient role as an outpatient.

In hospital, as well as being subordinate to medicine, midwifery is organized in a hierarchical manner designed for nursing. Within the hospital the hierarchy is ever present. The very reasons for the existence of hospitals – the centralization of medical expertise and equipment for maximum efficiency – to a large extent dictate the structure and, therefore, the problems of those within that structure. Freidson (1970b) looked at the professional dominance of medical expertise:

> *. . . the dominant profession stands in an entirely different structural relationship to the division of labour than does the subordinate profession. In essence, the difference reflects the existence of a hierarchy of institutional expertise . . . (which) can have the same effect upon the experience of the client as bureaucracy is said to have.*

Doctors have the power to define the situation. As Helen Roberts (1985) observed:

> *Doctor and patient normally agree that it is the doctor who defines the situation, and defines what is and what is not acceptable as appropriate for the patient to talk about.*

For the 'subordinate profession' too, the dominant profession has the power to define. Under the 1902 Act the midwife was, within the limits set by the Act, an independent practitioner in normal cases. Pregnancies were seen as normal until judged otherwise, though there was latterly some dispute as to whether the GP or midwife should make that judgement. As maternity care moved into hospital, the doctors' territory, the definer and the definition changed. All pregnancies fell under medical management and were seen as 'normal only in retrospect'. This phrase, originally used by obstetricians (Percival 1970), was soon to be used by the Central Midwives Board in their document *The Role of the Midwife* (CMB 1983). 'Medical science' had become the 'predominant source of the social constructs of the culture of childbirth' (Oakley 1993) as the Church had been in the Middle Ages. As part of that culture, midwives could not point out that 'Science is in this sense itself ideology; it is certainly not a matter of objective "fact" ' (Oakley 1993). By the logic of the medical scientific view, the midwife as a practitioner in her own right is defined out of existence and the hospital midwife's work is either obstetric nursing or what medical staff delegate as 'provisionally normal' (Cox 1982).

Technology, power and ideology

As men entered midwifery with their instruments, so the development of obstetrics saw the growth of obstetric technology. Whilst this has had benefits for women, it has profoundly affected power relationships. Brigitte Jordan (1987) analysed this as an anthropologist:

> *There is a hidden function of the tools of the trade that goes beyond their efficacy: it has to do with their symbolic function as indicators and enforcers of the social distribution of knowledge and power to act in childbirth. I suspect this symbolic function is partly responsible for the uncritical acceptance of the fetal monitor in high-technology settings.*

The growth of such technology has a profound effect on the woman and her attendants because information is now available to them that the mother did not provide. Ultrasound, for instance, enables doctors to assess the date the baby is due without reference to, or discussion of, the date of the mothers last menstrual period.

> *High technology, thus, draws in its wake a hierarchical distribution of knowledge and social authority that reflects the equally hierarchical social position of birth attendants in medicalised settings.*
>
> (Jordan 1987)

Thus the woman is on the professionals' territory surrounded by equipment that only they can interpret. The midwife often appears to take the role of machine minder.

Monitoring symbolizes a fundamental change in the obstetrics view of childbearing. It concerns all pregnancies and, compared with a statistical assessment of risk, normality seems a crude and possibly irrelevant concept. William Arney (1982, p. 85) has given us a rich analysis of obstetric knowledge and concludes:

> *Monitoring and surveillance deal with the problem of residual normalcy by ignoring it. Under this new regime no distinctions between normal and abnormal exist.*

Obstetrics has moved from a defined area of abnormal childbearing to a much wider view whilst at the same time accommodating demands from consumers for alternatives to the traditional medical model of birth.

> *The social organization of obstetrics extended outwards from the hospital over large areas, putting in place a flexible system of obstetrical alternatives as it went. Even so, every aspect of birth became more carefully controlled, a structure of control I call 'monitoring' was deployed across a greatly expanded obstetrical space.*
>
> (Arney 1982)

This ability to respond to a demand for flexibility whilst widening its area of power is a clear example of the 'chameleon-like qualities', the possession of which Saks (1992) sees as 'one of the reasons why the medical profession has been so successful to date in defending its interests'. Midwifery appears more like a well-trained domestic animal. No parallel, wide midwifery ideology exists beside the 'flexible system of obstetrical alternatives'. By Arney's analysis obstetrics has, in outgrowing its role of concern with the abnormal, threatened the adjacent role of concern with the normal. It could, therefore, be argued that the midwife has become, by default, a doctor's handmaiden, albeit a highly technological handmaiden. Perhaps this accounts for the increasing emphasis on teamwork when describing the midwife's role.

WHAT DO WOMEN WANT OF MIDWIVES?

There is no reason to assume that women are a homogeneous group but some themes run clearly through all the research on consumers' views on the maternity services. The most recurring of these themes are women's desire for information, continuity of care and to be treated with kindness (Reid and Garcia 1989). Research clearly shows that women want intelligible, consistent information with which to orientate themselves to their situation (Cartwright 1979, Oakley 1980, Kirke 1980). Surveys of the literature show appropriate information to be therapeutic (Reid and Garcia 1989). The desire for information runs through all stages of maternity care and is a crucial determinant of women's satisfaction with that care.

Though the need is apparent across all social groups, the giving of the right information in the right way for each individual woman is a very subtle skill. In Perkins' (1991) view:

Part of the explanation for midwives' failure to identify some women's needs lies with the difficulty they may have in expressing them. Women may lack practice in identifying their own needs, lack confidence in expressing them or have no expectations that the service will be interested in them anyway.

So midwives need well-developed skills in supporting women and listening to them before they can ascertain the needs of those many women who do not expect to be listened to. Such support can improve outcome (Oakley 1992). To give continuity of care and to treat women with kindness similarly require of midwives such skills in giving support and relating to all women, not just the articulate.

Our 'social support' midwives gave no clinical care. When asked what they had appreciated about this type of help, the mothers put the fact that 'she listened' first: eighty per cent of them said this was important.

(Oakley 1988)

Information, similarly, is not of value for its own sake. It enables women to orientate themselves to their situation, to weigh options and make choices. This is critically linked to the issue of control. In a large prospective study of child-bearing women, Green *et al.* (1988) concluded:

> *Women who feel informed about and involved in the management of labour and are able to retain some degree of 'external' as well as 'internal' control have better outcomes. The quality of staff care and how things are done are as important as what is done.*

These outcomes included postnatal emotional well-being and relationship with the baby, significant outcomes in view of the prevalence of postnatal depression. There are, of course, major dilemmas here, as Perkins (1991) said:

> *Asking women what they want used to be seen as a somewhat radical move, likely to undermine professional authority and professional judgement.*

The underlying dilemma is, however, deeper than the current fashion for consumer satisfaction which professions must accommodate in a market situation. Professions keep a specialist body of knowledge and control the consumer's construction of reality. Yet midwives are most successful both in their clients' view and in measurable postnatal outcome when they give information generously and when they empower women to feel in control of both themselves and their attendants.

A MIDWIFERY BODY OF KNOWLEDGE?

Before looking further at what midwives should do with their knowledge, it is useful to examine whether there is a unique midwifery body of knowledge and what is the working knowledge of midwives.

Knowledge of medicine and physiology

Midwives have a considerable amount of medical knowledge. No-one could now justify the early plans to limit this knowledge. Knowledge of physiology and of medicine is important for safe practice. There is also a body of knowledge and skill that has been delegated by medicine: 'innovations by doctors which once routinised are then delegated to nurses or other paramedical occupations' (Hughes 1971). In Jennifer Sleep's (1992) view:

. . . these newly acquired skills do not represent midwifery innovations prompted and directed by the needs of normally labouring women. Many are developed as a consequence of practitioners' frustration and consumer dissatisfaction and as such provide a means of reducing the time spent waiting for junior doctors to make and implement clinical decisions.

Dingwall *et al.* (1988) cautioned:

. . . this downward delegation of routinised, albeit skilled, medical tasks is at the expense of the (midwives') role as a spiritual, or in modern times, psychological support for the mother.

Not only is there less time, and less status, for the traditional support skills but the values of the delegating profession are implicit in the delegated tasks. In Schwartz's (1990) view:

One of the tasks assigned to the midwife in her new role as subcontractor to the (obstetric) engineering programme is to explain and to make mothers feel at ease with the new technologies.

Is this facilitating choice or ensuring acquiescence?

There is a deep dilemma in the knowledge in midwifery that comes from medicine. Medicine has taught us basic processes about normal childbearing and a great deal about the abnormal. It has also taught us important things about what to do when things go wrong. Medicine, however, whilst deeply involved with how actively to adjust deviations from the parameters it has established, has little study of the extent of normality and how normality can be retained. Yet there must also exist a vast area of study concerned with the nature of normal childbearing and factors that support or oppose that normality. A few doctors are involved in this study, but it is a vast area that extends far beyond the medical and pulls on many other disciplines. If midwives are concerned with normal childbearing surely this vast area of knowledge is one midwives must explore. There are signs of this in the way other disciplines are now involved in midwifery education.

Knowledge from midwifery research

A body of knowledge is beginning to be built from midwifery research. This has affected practice as shown in the great reduction in routine predelivery shaves and enemas. More importantly, in the words of a very experienced midwife researcher, this creates an attitude:

. . . fostering a greater sense of uncertainty in our approach to care: admitting that 'we do not know' can provide an impetus to the discovery and evaluation of ways in which practice can be improved.

(Sleep 1992)

Chalmers (1983) suggests that one of the features of scientific inquiry is its anti-authoritarian nature. Midwifery research is very new. Few aspects of midwifery have yet been researched. How does the questioning that must apply to all these areas fit with our claim to professionalism with its assumption of expert knowledge and status?

Knowledge from other midwives

There is, and always has been, knowledge and skill passed from midwife to midwife or student. The clinical part of midwifery education acknowledges this, though medical delegation and proceduralization have deeply affected the role models available. In the apprenticeship learning in midwifery, knowledge is transmitted in very different ways from the didactic methods of the classroom. We can all remember the hands that gently guided ours during our first deliveries.

To master the skill means to acquire expert body behaviour. . . . In a real sense, the knowledge is in the hands and transferred by the hands. It is truly embodied knowledge.

(Jordan 1989)

The importance of learning through touch and learning through socialization as an apprentice are relatively little acknowledged now education has become professionalized. In Jordan's view:

. . . the apprenticeship mode is good for learning how to do something, the didactic mode is for learning how to talk about doing something.

Perhaps this accounts for the many occasions (Kirkham 1989, Cutts 1993) when midwives say they do something in caring for women which they are not observed to do in practice.

In midwifery practice knowledge is often conveyed to students and to mothers by means of stories. 'I once looked after a woman who . . .' is an opening that always commands attention.

These stories, then, are packages of situated knowledge, knowledge which is not available abstractly, but is called up as the characteristics of the situation require it.

To acquire a store of appropriate stories and, even more importantly, to know what are appropriate occasions for telling them, is part of what it means to become a midwife.

(Jordan 1989)

It can be argued that such means of learning that do not involve statements of principle and which are relatively invisible give more power to the learner than does didactic teaching. Here the student is not required to verbalize what she accepts into her body of operating knowledge.

Midwifery skill can be most clearly seen where midwives have most autonomy, in tiny units and amongst community midwives. There are now attempts to make such skill more widely available by both research (Kirkham 1989) and by teaching students to observe and analyse role models. Ironically, some of our traditional midwifery skills are now coming into our formal body of knowledge through the work of women anthropologists such as Brigitte Jordan (1983, 1987, 1989). Such knowledge shows how much work is still needed to develop and reclaim this area of midwifery knowledge and to create the language and concepts needed for such development.

Knowledge from women

Midwives also gain knowledge from women: both individuals in their care and the women's organizations and publications concerning birth. In supporting women through childbearing we need to know how these events are subjectively experienced. For example, the transition between the first and second stage of labour is an unexpected and often unpleasant experience for many women and their partners. This stage of labour has no physical, measurable characteristics and therefore does not appear in medical texts. 'Transition' has, however, been described for many years in lay texts because it can be a very different experience from what precedes and follows it. Until we know that something is there, whether it is transition or the way a particular piece of technology may be perceived, we can neither prepare women for it nor help them through it. This is complex, as individuals have different experiences.

There is evidence that midwives gained knowledge through observation of women, which was only much later acknowledged by science. For instance, Leap and Hunter quote Elizabeth C (born 1905, trained as a midwife in Bradford in the 1930s, interviewed 1986):

I think myself that the system has a certain amount of sedative that it releases at a time like that (labour) ... I've seen people that just looked as if they were half

sozzled – and they hadn't had anything! . . . I think the body does release some-
thing into the system. If it's not interfered with by giving dope, it will work. But I
think when you interfere, it won't work then.

(Leap and Hunter 1993, p. 169)

This old lady accurately described the release of endorphins in undisturbed
labour. She did not know that research had discovered endorphins (Odent
1984). Without the ability to look through women's eyes, both intellectually
and in individual relationships, midwives are limited to seeing women through
the eyes of experts or through stereotypes. The early midwifery leaders' stereo-
type of working-class women must not be repeated. Yet research now shows
midwives stereotyping Asian women in their care (Bowler 1993). This could
be seen as more worrying than stereotyping by those far removed from the
client.

Here too midwives learn from stories. Every mother has her childbearing
story that she can tell for the rest of her life. The midwife needs to have the skill
to analyse a woman's story so as to find 'treasures buried entirely and hidden by
techniques which assume that all people share common constructs' (Stainton
Rogers 1991). The stories of a woman and her family's previous childbearing
are crucial knowledge for a midwife though they feature little in the standard
'previous obstetric history'. Yet the story tells much of its teller: her fears, hopes
and concerns, which the midwife must know to be 'with' this individual
woman. Similarly the midwife is part of the building of the new story and her
support can be of help as the new story crystallizes out in its early tellings. She
carries a duty to the mother to help her build a story that empowers her as a
parent. Such skill can more professionally be described as debriefing. The
important thing is that here, as in so much of midwifery, the mother is the doer
and the midwife the support.

Interpersonal skills

There is another area of midwifery knowledge and skill that concerns communication and interpersonal relations. Much of this is learnt in normal life.
Some of it is learnt from women in our care and some is learnt more
formally from other disciplines such as counselling. Ironically, as most midwives and all of our clients are women, learning communication skills in our
lives and from other women can enable us to fit neatly into the sexual division of labour in the obstetric hierarchy. There is progress, as shown on midwives' study days on assertiveness. More analysis is, however, needed to fuel
the insights into our knowledge and practice that make it open to change
and development.

Knowledge of giving support

There is a body of knowledge that shows that social support from midwives and others can improve outcomes in many aspects of maternity care (Oakley 1992). From this Oakley (1993) concludes:

> *Love is a scientific concept, and its effects on the health of childbearing women can be quantified . . . . Love – caring – is as important as science – technical knowledge, monitoring and intervention – in the maternity services today.*
>
> (Oakley 1993, pp. 76–7)

Midwives must have held this knowledge long before the technical knowledge existed and recent research on supportive care by social scientists and midwives (Evans 1991) has added to the traditional knowledge. Today there are problems in midwives' use of this knowledge. This first problem arises from the effects of what has been called the 'as if rule'. 'By treating all women as if they are about to become abnormal, obstetricians are inclined to make them so' (Oakley 1993). Given the power of obstetricians it is not surprising that this inclination is so often more powerful than midwives' ability to 'encourage the normal'. Oakley is sure that the 'goals of satisfying mothers and producing healthy babies, which are so often deemed by obstetricians to be at odds with one another, are in reality the same goal' (Oakley 1993, p. 77). Ironically, when this is realized, the response of the dominant profession is to define this knowledge into its own professional sphere. This was demonstrated in the 1960s by the incorporation of women's demands for less dehumanizing care into the new technical language of maternal infant bonding (Arney 1982). This irony of professional power is clearly demonstrated by the medical innovators of *Active Management of Labour* who stress, as part of their medically controlled management of labour, that:

> *The nurse (sic) must appreciate that her primary duty to the mother is to provide the emotional support so badly needed at this critical time and not simply to record vital signs in a detached clinical manner.*
>
> (O'Driscoll *et al.* 1993)

As part of this medical package 'a prior guarantee is given to every pregnant woman who attends this hospital that she will have a personal nurse (sic) through the whole labour', a promise many midwifery managers elsewhere would find hard to keep and which in Dublin 'would not be feasible unless the duration of labour was restricted' (p. 94). Thus basic midwifery care becomes part of a medical system which has the power to give guarantees and the knowledge concerning supporting women is seen as part of a medical repertoire of control which includes 'the need to keep every woman in labour on a tight emotional rein' (p. 92). It is concluded (p. 101) that:

> *Among the many benefits which have accrued from the active management of labour, none is more gratifying to observe than the boost given to the professional status of midwives in this hospital.*

Thus the midwife is given status only within a very tightly controlled medical system and the benefits of supportive midwifery care provide further proof of the benefits of the total obstetric management package. The *Active Management of Labour* package is fascinating because, by British obstetric standards, it contains relatively active, though closely prescribed, roles for midwife and mother within a 'clear chain of command, which can be seen to function with military efficiency but with a human face' (p. 103). Normal labour as the midwife's concern is seen as history for:

> *Nowadays, senior registrars are cast firmly in the role of obstetric physicians, rather than surgeons, with most emphasis on the conduct of labour in normal cases.*
>
> (O'Driscoll *et al.* 1993, p. 98)

This is the situation, which Arney (1982) equates with Foucault's (1977) panoptican, where all is constantly surveyed and controlled by those in authority.

There is a further irony that, as the midwife's professional role comes to constrain her role 'with woman', the role of supportive companion to the childbearing woman is being developed as a separate role. This started in America with the 'doula' supporter for breastfeeding women (Raphael 1976). As labour became more technical the importance of support in labour became more clear. Research in several countries has shown that a supportive female companion in labour can improve the outcome of labour in many measurable ways (Klaus *et al.* 1993). 'Doula' labour supporters are now being trained in this country but the doula role is seen as a separate role from that of the midwife, whose organizational constraints stop her from giving continuous support. All the women who benefit from a doula's care will also be in the care of another woman, the midwife. The need for a doula suggests to me that midwifery has lost its way whatever it has gained in status.

We must not, therefore, assume that all is progress in midwifery knowledge. Knowledge that midwives hold may not be used in practice or may be used by others as shown above. With social change some knowledge is also lost. This is clear in breastfeeding where midwives:

> *. . . know less and (are) less confident in breastfeeding than their illliterate grand-mothers because their training (devoted in large part to artificial feeding) will have destroyed their unconsciously absorbed knowledge.*
>
> (Palmer 1993)

Jacono (1993) claims more generally that 'some things which ought to be intuitively obvious about caring have been lost' following professionalization and routinization of caring roles. Knowledge is socially constructed and changes as society changes. We can, however, develop our awareness of this so that we can make judgements as to what we value enough to endeavour to retain. The research skills are available if we have the political will to do this.

There appears, therefore, to be a midwifery body of knowledge, still in need of much development, which is drawn from many disciplines. The most promising areas in which it is developing scarcely fit the professional model. Indeed, this model may be responsible for important losses in knowledge. To claim this knowledge as exclusive sounds highly professional and very arrogant. Who do we seek to exclude? If we exclude the women we serve we also cut off a major source of knowledge. Is it possible for midwifery knowledge to be grounded in and available to the women we serve, or must we accept that:

> *Knowledge based on complex machinery and high technology is in principle not communicable. No amount of good will on caregivers' parts could possibly solve this problem.*
>
> (Jordan 1987, p. 39)

If this is so we may have attained the mystic of professionalism but can we claim to be with women or even working in women's best interests? Clearly a crucial issue is how we use our knowledge.

MIDWIFERY PROCESSES FOR USING KNOWLEDGE TO ACHIEVE OUTCOMES

Institutional procedures and routines

Midwifery is full of examples of knowledge and skill becoming fossilized into procedures. Schon (1987) described proceduralization as 'attempts to reduce professional practice to a set of absolute, precise, implementable procedures, coupled with controls'. By 'control' he meant 'how to get people to do what you think they ought to do', which leads to 'the multiplication of systems of control so that when things go wrong the response is to increase and improve procedures'. We have all worked in places where practice is hedged about by policies and procedures, many of which date from disasters in the history of that unit rather than being grounded in research.

Such a setting may help individuals to cope with anxiety (Menzies 1970) but it can also 'serve to confine and limit the actions of the clinician, leaving little scope for professional judgement, skill, wisdom or creativity' (Sleep 1992). Sadly, research shows midwives believing they still exercise clinical judgement when thus confined (Henderson 1984), a major delusion in the I/T ratio.

Personal procedures and routines

Beneath such proceduralization are deeper problems. 'In order to retain a sense of control we need sameness and predictability in our daily experience' (Campbell 1984). We therefore generalize and create routines for our own protection. Yet for each childbearing woman, her experience is unique and for the midwife to offer really appropriate care she must step beyond generalization to be with this particular woman. In professional life 'the *pain* of keeping to knowledge of the particular is rarely sufficiently noticed' (Campbell 1984). We cannot do this where we ourselves feel threatened.

Beyond the shelter of professional routine, care of individual excellence can be achieved. Support for the practitioner is crucial or the cost of leaving that shelter would soon be too great to bear.

Well-worn habits

We also see today many strategies for using midwifery knowledge to achieve a desired outcome which are rooted in our history.

Deference and working by proxy

A classic example of this is 'the doctor–nurse game', first described 30 years ago:

> *The object of the game is as follows: the nurse is to be bold, have initiative and be responsible for making significant recommendations, while at the same time she must appear passive. This must be done in such a manner so as to make her recommendations appear to be initiated by the physician.*
>
> (Stein 1967)

Looking at the 'game' again in 1990, Stein *et al.* saw some changes as a result of improved nurse education, social change and the development of the 'stubborn rebel' within nursing. This picture rings very true to midwives in the basic 'game' and recent changes. Kitzinger *et al.* (1990) observed from their research:

> *Almost every midwife could immediately provide a list of tactics of 'how to get the SHO to do what you want'. It was as if they had all read the same manual on 'Gaining SHOs Compliance' . . . the end result was that they were involved in a great deal of what we chose to call 'hierarchy maintenance work'.*

Working 'by proxy' through men was essential for our unenfranchized fore-mothers. We still do it, though they won for us the vote and society and even medicine have changed. Perhaps the increasing numbers of non-nurses now entering midwifery will be less inclined to work in this way. Yet it is part of female culture, and as a pre-registration midwifery student observed to me when studying the 'game' recently: 'Every married woman does that'.

If we work by deference and proxy we ensure that at best the more power-ful profession is 'right'. As we engage in 'hierarchy maintenance work' we also demonstrate to mothers our humble role in the hierarchy, which in turn implies that they are even more powerless.

Scapegoating

Attempts to raise our professional standing have often led to scapegoating within midwifery. This is shown above with *bona fide* midwives and later part-time working-class midwives despite the evidence of good outcome from these groups. Hopefully the advent of large numbers of non-nurse midwives and our growing self-awareness will prevent these historical patterns from being repeated. A cynic could, however, see a similar process in moves to raise the academic level of midwifery training without evaluation of the previous 'lower' academic qualifications.

In a relatively powerless position professionally it is easy for the midwife to fall back on her expert role relative to the client who has even less power.

> *The more the specialised knowledge of the caregiver increases and becomes evident in interaction, the more the power of the client decreases.*
>
> (DeVries 1989)

'Problems in the midwifery profession and the maternity services are thus acted out upon women' (Isherwood 1992). This is clearly neither 'with woman' nor therapeutic but is a very real professional temptation. Indeed, the professional role of the midwife leaves a very fine line between managing care and leaving the woman feeling that her experience has been managed to the point of alienation. Elizabeth Davis (1981) sees this as destroying the essence of midwifery which is being humble and paying attention. The many definitions of professionalism do not mention being humble.

So our professional past and present are full or ironies. Aspiring to professional status, yet surrounded by powerful interests, midwifery has tended to act out of insecurity: creating scapegoats and lagging behind major movements for reform. For a small group powerful alliances have tended to require deference, indeed without its skilful exercise in Victorian times midwifery would not now exist in this country. Low status within the hierarchy, increasing our insecurity, can lead to arrogance with clients.

LOOKING TO THE FUTURE

As we look to the future we are inevitably affected by our past. The process of professionalization has created dilemmas in three key sets of relationships. It is perhaps useful to look to the future in terms of these relationships.

Relationships within midwifery

Surrounded by more powerful groups, and intimately involved with life and death, midwives are in a vulnerable position. Seeking to be professional does not allow us to acknowledge that vulnerability and midwifery has therefore experienced considerable insecurity in the past 100 years. This insecurity, together with aspirations to higher status, has led to scapegoating and a culture within midwifery that is quick to blame but slow to praise or appreciate midwives' achievements. Such a situation is exacerbated by the constant changes in health care of recent years.

Such insecurity at all levels in midwifery can cause rigidity and lead to change being seen as a threat. For instance, a recent report on team midwifery (Wraight *et al.* 1993) tellingly observed:

Many senior midwives and medical staff opposed the change since the need to devolve responsibility, for the total care of the woman, down to the team midwife caused them anxiety.

In such a situation of insecurity reflection on the shortcomings of our practice is often blocked. This is sadly clear to those outside midwifery who try to work with us. Gabrielle Palmer (1993) observed of her work on breastfeeding:

I worry a lot about the feelings of (midwives) and go round in circles trying to be tactful when stating harsh truths. Why? Because I know there is no system of support for their wounded feelings and often denial is their only defence.

Oakley and Houd (1990, p. 83) list the types of defence mechanisms midwives develop, all of which limit development and sensitivity in future practice. They conclude:

One implication of the midwife's vulnerability is that midwives need their own support systems, and perhaps expert therapeutic help, to understand and work through their experiences . . . . They need to talk about fear and insecurity – for example, in connection with responsibility and the risk of being accused of having made a mistake. This is difficult in the hierarchical system of a hospital.

Available sources of support are embedded in that hierarchy. A midwife seeking support from her local branch of the Royal College of Midwives may well find its officers are all her managers at work, and her supervisor of midwives is also her manager. Clearly other support systems are needed. There are some cheering moves as in the setting up of staff support systems and the growing emphasis on the need for personal support systems in midwifery education. Much more needs to be done.

Midwifery supervision has changed from the punitive system earlier this century but it is significant that there is still no appeal against supervisory decisions. We need to reach a point where supervision is sought as an opportunity for individuals to receive support and plan how to improve their practice in a safe setting. There is much to be learnt here from supervision in other fields such as counselling (Hawkins and Shohet 1989). Support of all sorts is essential if we are to achieve the confidence as midwives to outgrow the scapegoat responses of professionalism. Then we can develop the flexibility to find an appropriate balance between our need to feel in control of our work and each woman's need to feel in control of her experience.

Research can also be used to improve midwives' confidence and self-esteem. Are we familiar with the abundant evidence which shows that 'midwives manage normal pregnancy as well as, if not better than physicians'? Yet 'the general rule appears to be that midwives do less than they are allowed' (Oakley and Houd 1990). So often research is experienced by midwives as something used to bludgeon them to change. Used appropriately it can increase midwives' confidence and our level of analytical skill concerning our practice. We can then develop the skills to practise from secure basic principles; knowing why we act and to what end. Surely this is the only way to practise safely.

We also need much more research on midwifery practice so that we can learn systematically from existing excellent role models and from which we can develop theory. The resulting theory may apply such concepts as 'skilled companionship' and 'moderated love' (Campbell 1984) to the existing knowledge on social support in maternity care. Such concepts call for great skill and caring which require the carer to be in all senses close to the mother. Such ideas stand in contrast to the divide between the mother and the carer that the enhanced status of professionalism implies.

With increasingly appropriate knowledge and support we can address the issue of midwifery management. Structures need to be changed. More woman-focused care is likely to be less hierarchical but vision is needed to start such processes of change. There are now examples of how this can be done with the ownership of the midwives involved for the immediate benefit of those we serve (Davies 1992).

Relationships with women

Women need midwives with highly developed skills because:

> *First the exclusion from childbirth of autonomous midwifery restricts the options available to childbearing women and inevitably promotes the definition of childbearing as a pathological medicalised process. Second, while the dominant myth of the age is that official medicine is scientific and effective, whereas lay alternatives are not, it is often the case that official medicine is neither effective nor scientific, while alternative forms of care can be both.*
>
> (Oakley and Houd 1990, p. 114)

Midwives need to be confident, knowledgeable and articulate to make these things known and to act upon them. We need a clear strong leadership voice to state these issues and lobby for the funds to achieve excellent maternity care. Appropriate alliances are crucial but we will not gain them by deference.

Midwives need to listen to women, as individuals and in general terms, in order to further our common interests. Continuity of care can be one way towards this. This is something long wanted by childbearing women that midwifery organizations have more recently come to champion. The recommendations of the Winterton Report (HMSO 1992) and *Changing Childbirth* (Department of Health 1993) provide a unique opportunity. These are the first government documents on maternity care in which women's experiences have been central and midwives have been seen as 'with women'. There is potential in the move from fragmented care to sustained relationships with women to transform midwifery practice (Flint 1993). We can really develop the art of being with women and small teams working as equals can transform the hierarchies in which we work.

There are many team midwifery schemes at present but is midwifery being transformed? In *Mapping Team Midwifery*, Wraight *et al.* (1993) looked at many schemes and concluded:

> *It appears that few team midwifery schemes are organised in such a way as to maximise those features most strongly associated with higher levels of continuity of care.*

Perhaps this is not surprising if our aim in terms of mothers' experience is lost sight of in our concentration on the mechanics of providing the service. In Curell's (1990) view:

> *When continuity of care is discussed in relation to the maternity services it is primarily describing characteristics of the working life of the care providers not the total experience of the woman . . . descriptions of 'continuity of care' are descriptions of the way professionals organise their work, not a description or definition of the nature or quality of any care that may be given within that particular organisational framework.*

If we could change our focus 'away from the caregiver and towards the woman herself' (Curell 1990) then clarity of aim could be followed by planning the means to achieve that aim. Many team midwifery schemes have been abandoned for organizational reasons but 'I have yet to hear client dissatisfaction quoted as a cause for abandoning team care' (Kroll 1993).

Clearly midwives must support those they exist to be with. The issue of advocacy is, however, more complex. Women are not a homogeneous group; indeed, interests can conflict within that group. Midwives often need to speak for those with least voice and greatest need rather than simply support the articulate. This is to do with enabling women to take the control that improves outcome not controlling them as professionals. Ruth Ashton, general secretary of the Royal College of Midwives, states:

> *. . . midwives cannot be women's advocates because their professional status, their skills and their knowledge, by definition, set them apart from women in general . . . a midwife might find it difficult to support a woman who either demanded care that was unsafe or that would lead to the midwife transgressing her code of practice.*
>
> (Ashton 1992)

Perhaps we need to examine more closely what is meant by safety. There can be few midwives who have not given care for the safety of staff rather than clients in a climate of defensive medicine. When we really understand her concept of safety and acknowledge that nothing is completely safe, does any mother want care that threatens herself or her baby? Or is this a category of mothers created in the process of debate?

'Consumer empowerment mechanisms' (Ashton 1992) are not without dilemmas. Consumer choice is not in itself empowering because the provider defines the options from which choice can be made and the consumer may wish to choose something completely different. In these circumstances do we blame her or change the system to accommodate her? Surely childbearing women are engaged in the ultimate productive act rather than passive consumers of health care. Is it possible for our expertise to set us only far enough apart from women to have a firm footing from which to give them support whilst still being near enough to speak for those who cannot be heard?

Alliance with mothers does not mean that midwives do not have their own needs. In Gabrielle Palmer's (1993) words, 'if you are to care about mothers and babies, first care about yourselves'. Can we learn ways of looking after ourselves that do not create a barrier between us and those in our care? Can we learn to accept support from the women we serve from whom we gain so much? This problem is fundamental for all women carers, solutions are likely also to be held in common. Exploration of this area could be immensely strengthening.

Relations with other professionals

We have a traditional relationship with medicine that was enabling for doctors. We now need to develop relationships that are enabling for midwives and women.

The recent growth in midwifery-led care is very important and not without historical irony. Midwives are a relatively inexpensive commodity, especially when separated from the expenses of hospital stay. There is great potential here to develop our skills and expertise but women's needs and experiences must be central. Perhaps alongside more home births and early transfer home we need to campaign for more home helps.

We need the strength to ensure that our skills are not subsumed within medical knowledge and then straitjacketed by medicine. This calls for strong leadership in alliance with women. We must ensure that research which shows how support improves outcome is widely implemented. We also need to ensure that our skills are available to all women. Not all women experience normal childbearing and many who do also want to make some use of high technology services in, for example, antenatal screening. Yet what women want of midwives, and the skills in relating and communicating that midwives are developing, are relevant to all women not just the normal. We need therefore to develop our skills in communication so that we can empower women in the presence of other professions and of technology. We live in a technical age. With a mid-wife's support during labour and a midwife's voice in equipment design surely it is possible for a monitor to be as immediately useful to a mother in labour as her microwave or video is to her at home.

If we really develop the skills of being 'with woman', we have much to offer medicine and related professions as many studies (Cartwright 1964) have shown communication failure to be patients' most commonly voiced criticism of health care in general. The values implicit in professionalization have led us to take on the values of the dominant profession emphasizing technical skill. 'When this happened the "love" part of the work was lost' (Smith 1992). We need now to develop the 'emotional labour' of care.

> *Rather than being a soft option, it is a fundamental necessity. For those who wish to concern themselves with scientific proof, this can be demonstrated from published studies examining the effects of social support as distinct from clinical care.*
> (Oakley 1993, p. 77)

It is historically ironic that there is much here that we can learn from nursing research (James 1989, Smith 1992).

We have come a long way by varying and often devious routes. Now we can learn from the patterns of that past. The decisions we make are political deci-sions because they state our priorities and determine our alliances. Professionalism, like the Victorian attitudes that achieved the 1902 Act, can only get us so far. We can and must go further. As Ehrenreich and English concluded after surveying our history:

> *We must never confuse professionalism with expertise. Expertise is something to work for and to share: professionalism is – by definition – elitist and exclusive, sexist, racist and classist.*
> (Ehrenreich and English 1973)

Indeed professionalism can now be seen as 'positively damaging to health' (Oakley 1984), not least the health of midwives.

We know what women want of us and how we can improve outcome for them. We need to view safety in the long-term context of the emotional well-being of families. This suggests our service must be women-centred. We need to generate the strength to make knowledge and control available to women despite the pressures on us to retain knowledge and power. We need the humility to learn from social scientists, doulas and many, many others. Thus we can increase the knowledge available for women not hoard our knowledge of women. If we thus give women our attention, we face the dilemma of caring and integrity for ourselves and for childbearing women. This is a female carers' dilemma for which a new model is needed. That model should not be static and defensive but dynamic and giving. We can create that model together.

A profession of belief as to where we stand and who we serve may be more useful to midwifery now than a claim to professional status.

REFERENCES

Arney, W.R. (1982) *Power and the Profession of Obstetrics*, Chicago: University of Chicago Press.

Ashton, R. (1992) 'Who Can Speak for Women?', *Nursing Times*, Vol. 88, No. 29, p. 70.

Bourdillon, H. (1988) *Women as Healers*, Cambridge: Cambridge University Press.

Bowler, I.M.W. (1993) Stereotypes of women of Asian descent in midwifery: some evidence, *Midwifery* **9:** 7–16.

Campbell, A.V. (1984) *Moderated Love: A Theology of Professional Care*, London: SPCK.

Campbell, J.M. (1924) *Maternal Mortality Associated With Childbearing*, London: HMSO.

Cartwright, A. (1964) *Human Relations and Hospital Care*, London: Routledge and Kegan Paul.

Cartwright, A. (1979) *The Dignity of Labour*, London: Tavistock.

Central Midwives Board (1983) *The Role Of The Midwife*, Norwich: Hymns Ancient and Modern.

Chalmers, I. (1983) Scientific enquiry and authoritarianism in perinatal care and education. *Birth* **10:** 151–6.

Chalmers, I., Enkin, M. and Keirse, M.J.N.C. (eds) (1989) *Effective Care in Pregnancy and Childbirth*, Oxford: Oxford University Press.

Chamberlain, M. (1981) *Old Wives Tales*, London: Virago Press.

Cox, C. (1982) 'Where Are We Now?', *Midwives Chronicle*, January, pp. 3–6.

Curell, R. (1990) The organisation of midwifery care. In Alexander, J., Levy, V. and Roch, S. (eds) *Antenatal Care: A Research-Based Approach*, London: Macmillan.

Cutts, D.E. (1993) Counselling: Midwives Do Not Do What They Say Or Think They Do. Paper to ICM Conference, Vancouver, 1993.

Davies, J. (1992) The role of the midwife in the 1990s. In Chard, T. and Richards, M.P.M. (eds) *Obstetrics in the 1990s: Current Controversies*, London: MacKeith Press.

Davis, C. (1983) Professional strategies as time- and culture-bound: American and British nursing circa 1893. In Langeman, E.C. (ed.) *Nursing History: New Perspectives. New Possibilities*, New York: Teachers College Press.

Davis, E. (1981) *Heart and Hands. A Midwife's Guide to Pregnancy and Birth*, Berkley, California: Celestial Arts.

Department of Health (1993) *Changing Childbirth: Report of the Expert Maternity Group*, London: HMSO.

DeVries, R.G. (1989) Caregivers in pregnancy and childbirth. In Chalmers, I., Enkin, M. and Keirse, M.J.N.C. (eds) *Effective Care in Pregnancy and Childbirth*, Oxford: Oxford University Press.

Dingwall, R. and Lewis, P. (1983) *The Sociology of Professions: Lawyers, Doctors and Others*, London: Macmillan.

Dingwall, R., Rafferty, A.M. and Webster, C. (1988) *An Introduction to the Social History of Nursing*, London: Routledge, Chapman and Hall.

Donnison, J. (1977) *Midwives and Medical Men*, London: Heinemann.

Ehrenreich, B. and English, D. (1973) *Witches, Midwives and Nurses: A History of Women Healers*, New York: The Feminist Press, Glass Mountain Pamphlet.

Elliot, P. (1972) *The Sociology of Professions*, New York: Macmillan.

Etzioni, A. (ed.) (1969) *The Semi-Professions and their Organisation*, New York: Free Press.

Evans, F.B. (1991) The Newcastle Community Midwifery Care Project: the evaluation of the project. In Robinson, S. and Thomson, A.M. (eds) *Midwives, Research and Childbirth Vol. 2*, London: Chapman and Hall.

Flint, C. (1993) *Midwifery Teams and Caseloads*, Oxford: Butterworth Heinemann.

Foucault, M. (1977) *Discipline and Punish*, Harmondsworth: Penguin.

Freidson, E. (1970a) *Profession of Medicine*, New York: Dodd Mead and Co.

Freidson, E. (1970b) *Professional Dominance: The Social Structure of Medical Care*, Chicago: Aldine.

Green, J.M., Coupland, V. and Kitzinger, J.V. (1988) *Great Expectations: A Prospective Study of Women's Expectations and Experiences of Childbirth*, Cambridge: Child Care and Development Group, University of Cambridge.

Gregory, A. (ed.) (1923) *The Midwife: Her Book*, London: Frowde and Hodder and Stoughton.

Hawkins, P. and Shohet, R. (1989) *Supervision and the Helping Professions*, Milton Keynes: Open University Press.

Heagerty, B.V. (1990) *Gender and Professionalization: the Struggle for British Midwifery, 1900–1936*, unpublished thesis, Michigan State University, 1990 (copy in Royal College of Midwives Library, London).

Henderson, C. (1984) Influences and interactions surrounding the midwife's decision to rupture the membranes. In *Research and the Midwife Conference Proceedings*.

HMSO (1892) *Report from the Select Committee on the Registration of Midwives, House of Commons*, London: HMSO.

HMSO (1992) *Parliamentary Select Committee on Health: Second Report on the Maternity Services*, London: HMSO.

Hughes, E.C. (1971) *The Sociological Eye*, Chicago: Aldine.

Illich, I., Zola, I.K., McKnight, J., Caplan, J. and Shaiken, H. (1977) *Disabling Professions*, New York: Marion Boyars.

Isherwood, K.M. (1992) 'Are British Midwives "With Women"? – The Evidence', *Midwifery Matters*, Vol. 54, Autumn, pp. 14–17.

Jacono, B.J. (1993) Caring is loving, *Journal of Advanced Nursing* **18**: 192–4.

James, N. (1989) Emotional labour, skills and work in the social regulation of feeling, *Sociological Review* **37**: 15–42.

Jamous, H. and Peloille, B. (1970) Professions or self-perpetuating systems? In Jackson, J.A. (ed.) *Professions and Professionalisation*, Cambridge: Cambridge University Press.

Johnson, T. (1972) *Professions and Power*, London: Macmillan.

Jordan, B. (1983) *Birth in Four Cultures*, Montreal: Eden Press.

Jordan, B. (1987) 'The Hut and the Hospital: Information, Power and Symbolism in the Artifacts of Birth', *Birth*, Vol. 14, No. 1, March, pp. 36–40.

Jordan, B. (1989) Cosmopolitical obstetrics: some insights from the training of traditional midwives, *Social Science and Medicine* 28: 925–44.

Kirke, P.N. (1980) Mothers' views of obstetric care, *British Journal of Obstetrics and Gynaecology* **87**: 1029–33.

Kirkham, M.J. (1989) Midwives and information-giving during labour. In Robinson, S. and Thomson, A.M. (eds) *Midwives, Research and Childbirth Vol. 1*, London: Chapman and Hall.

Kitzinger, J., Green, J. and Coupland, V. (1990) Labour relations: midwives and doctors on the labour ward. In Garcia, J., Kilpatrick, R. and Richards, M. (eds) *The Politics of Maternity Care*, Oxford: Clarendon Press.

Klaus, M.L., Kennell, J.H. and Klaus, P.H. (1993) *Mothering the Mother*, Reading, Massachusetts: Addison-Wesley.

Kroll, D. (1993) 'The Name of the Game – Team Midwifery Now', *Modern Midwife*, May/June, pp. 26–8.

Larkin, G. (1983) *Occupational Monopoly and Modern Medicine*, London: Tavistock.

Larson, M. (1977) *The Rise of Professionalism*, California: University of California Press.

Leap, N. and Hunter, B. (1993) *The Midwife's Tale*, London: Scarlet Press.

Llewelyn Davies, M. (ed.) (1977) *Life As We Have Known It: By Cooperative Working Women*, London: Virago.

Menzies, I. (1970) *The Functioning of Social Systems and a Defense Against Anxiety*, London: Tavistock Institute of Human Relations.

Midwives Record (1910) Can be found in the British Museum, London.

Ministry of Health (1929) *Report of the Departmental Committee on the Training and Employment of Midwives*, London: HMSO.

Nursing Notes can be found in the Royal College of Midwives Library, London.

Oakley, A. (1976) Wisewoman and Medicine Man: changes in the management of childbirth. In Oakley, A. and Mitchell, J. (eds) *The Rights and Wrongs of Women*, Harmondsworth: Penguin.

Oakley, A. (1980) *Women Confined: Towards a Sociology of Childbirth*, Oxford: Martin Robertson.

Oakley, A. (1984) 'What Price Professionalism? *Nursing Times*, Vol. 80, No. 50, pp. 24–7.

Oakley, A. (1988) 'Who Cares For Women? Science and Love in Midwifery Today', William Powell Memorial Lecture 1988, published in Oakley, A. (1993).

Oakley, A. (1992) *Social Support and Motherhood*, Oxford: Blackwell.

Oakley, A. (1993) *Essays on Women, Medicine and Health*, Edinburgh: Edinburgh University Press.

Oakley, A. and Houd, S. (1990) *Helpers in Childbirth: Midwifery Today*, London: Hemisphere on behalf of WHO Regional Office for Europe.

Odent, M. (1984) *Birth Reborn*, London: Souvenir Press.

O'Driscoll, K., Meagher, D. and Boylan, P. (1993) *Active Management of Labour*. London: Mosby.

Paget, R. (1901) Quoted, courtesy of RCM archives, in Heagerty, B.V. (1990) *Gender and Professionalization: the Struggle for British Midwifery*, unpublished PhD thesis, Michigan State University.

Palmer, G. (1993) 'Who Helps the Professional With Breast Feeding?' *Midwives Chronicle*, Vol. 106; No. 1264, May, pp. 147–56.

Parkin, F. (1979) *Marxism and Class Theory: A Bourgeoise Critique*, London: Tavistock.

Parry, N. and Parry, J. (1976) *The Rise of the Medical Profession*, London: Croom Helm.

Percival, R. (1970) 'Management of Normal Labour', *The Practitioner*, Vol. 1221, March, p. 204.

Perkins, E.R. (1991) 'What Do Women Want: Asking Consumers' Views', *Midwives Chronicle*, Vol. 104, No. 1247, pp. 347–54.

Raphael, D. (1976) *The Tender Gift: Breastfeeding*, New York: Schocken Books.

Reid, M. and Garcia, J. (1989) Women's views of care during pregnancy and childbirth. In Chalmers, I., Enkin, M. and Keirse, M.J.N.C. (eds) *Effective Care In Pregnancy and Childbirth*, Oxford: Oxford University Press.

Roberts, H. (1985) *The Patients Patients: Women and Their Doctors*, London: Pandora.

Saks, M. (ed.) (1992) *Alternative Medicine in Britain*, Oxford: Clarendon.

Schon, D.L. (1987) Changing patterns of inquiry in work and living, *Journal of the Royal Society of Arts* **135:** 225–37.

Schwarz, E.W. (1990) The engineering of childbirth: a new obstetric programme as reflected in British obstetric textbooks, 1969–1980. In Garcia, J., Kilpatrick, R. and Richards, M. (eds) *The Politics of Maternity Care*, Oxford: Clarendon.

Seligman, M.E.P. (1975) *Helplessness: On Depression, Development and Death*, San Francisco: Friedman.

Simpson, R.I. and Simpson, I.H. (1969) Women and bureaucracy in the semi-professions. In Etzioni, A. (ed.) *The Semi-Professions and Their Organisation*, New York: Free Press.

Sleep, J. (1992) Research and the practice of midwifery, *Journal of Advanced Nursing* 17: 1465–71.

Smith, F.B. (1979) *The People's Health 1830–1910*, London: Croom Helm.

Smith, P. (1992) *The Emotional Labour of Nursing*, London: Macmillan.

Stainton Rogers, W. (1991) *Explaining Health and Illness: An Exploration of Diversity*, London: Harvester Wheatsheaf.

Stein, L. (1967) The doctor–nurse game, *Archives of General Psychiatry* **16:** 698–703.

Stein, L., Watts, D. and Howell, T. (1990) The doctor–nurse game revisited, *New England Journal of Medicine* **332:** 546–9.

Sullivan, D.A. and Weitz, R. (1989) *Labour Pains: Modern Midwives and Home Birth*, New Haven and London: Yale University Press.

Tew, M. (1978) The case against hospital deliveries: the statistical evidence. In Kitzing, S and Davis, J. (eds) *The Place of Birth*, Oxford: Oxford University Press.

Tew, M. (1986) 'The Practice of Birth Attendants and the Safety of Birth', *Midwifery*, Vol. 2, No. 1, March, pp. 3–10.

Titmuss, R. (1968) *Commitment to Welfare*, London: Allen and Unwin.

Weitz, R. and Sullivan, D. (1985) Licensed lay midwifery and the medical model of childbirth, *Sociology of Health and Illness* 7: 36–54.

Witz, A. (1992) *Professions and Patriarchy*, London: Routledge.

Wraight, A., Ball, J., Seccombe, I. and Stock, J. (1993) *Mapping Team Midwifery*, A Report to the Department of Health, Sussex: Institute of Manpower Studies, Sussex University.

9

Women and Midwives: Turning the Tide

Mary Newburn and Eileen Hutton

People come to us not so we will care for them but so we will help them care for themselves.

(lay midwife quoted in Katz Rothman 1982)

The seeds of a childbirth movement were sewn in this country in the late 1950s. It was a time when the place of birth was moving from home to hospital. Specialist obstetricians were becoming increasingly involved in the care of healthy women with normal pregnancies while district midwives and general practitioners (GPs) were seeing fewer women for the whole of their care. Discussion about birth was considered taboo (Allen 1990), so there were few opportunities for talking about what happened. Many women were unsure about the process of having a baby and afraid of labour. Those who were determined to find out often turned to medical textbooks. As recently as 1970, Angela Young – who later joined the National Childbirth Trust (NCT), organizing local study days, representing local women on the community health council and developing birth education in schools – described how she felt when she was expecting her baby: 'I wasn't afraid it was going to be painful, I was afraid it was going to be agony'.

Gradually, social attitudes to birth have changed. Bookstands are now full of magazines for expectant women. Films and photographs of births are commonplace. Following the parliamentary all-party *Maternity Services* report (Health Select Committee 1992), and *Changing Childbirth* (Department of Health 1993), the report of the Expert Maternity Group, even the medical press is more likely to discuss birth from the mother's point of view. A recent edition of a journal for GPs devoted a page to detailed accounts by two women of giving birth. Both had their baby in water. One of them, herself a GP, had prepared for the birth by learning hypnotherapy (Halle 1994). This kind of reporting would once have been unheard of.

The climate and provision of maternity care has come a long way. This chapter looks at the contribution women have made, and the organizations that have represented them. The authors have talked to women with a long-standing interest in maternity care and have drawn on published and unpublished material, particularly NCT papers. The chapter explores the policies and strategies of the NCT and other maternity organizations, considering the part they have played in influencing the quality of information, care and support available to women and the role of midwives in providing care. Finally, it suggests that organizations representing mothers and midwives now share the view that maternity care should be women–centred and provided by a small number of familiar midwives, with known doctors providing medical care if it is needed.

THE CHILDBIRTH MOVEMENT

In numerous countries throughout the post–war, Western world concerned individuals, women, parents, midwives, obstetricians and others have protested against the prevailing way of birth and advocated an alternative approach. Some of the influential early writing and the grouping together of individuals around a common cause began in the 1950s and grew slowly and quietly throughout the 1960s. During that time, awareness was spread through community networks. However, it was not until the 1970s, when feminism and consumerism became forces in their own right, that the childbirth movement began to have power of numbers and sufficient sway to influence change dramatically.

Over the years there have been differences of emphasis and of reasoning within the movement, but there has also been broad agreement. Concern focused on the demeaning circumstances in which women gave birth and experienced the first hours and days of motherhood in hospital. As critical analysis of maternity care has grown, commentators have suggested that the professionals providing care have in fact been preoccupied – though not necessarily consciously – with objectives separate from meeting the needs of mothers, babies or the wider family. In particular, there has been a widespread questioning of the medicalization and centralization of maternity care. A parallel concern has been expressed over the way the midwife's role has been transformed from independent practitioner to obstetric nurse (Donnison 1988, Kitzinger 1988, Oakley and Houd 1990).

Generally, there has been a wish to see more holistic care focusing on human, social values rather than medical ones. There has been a desire for clear information and emotional support as well as appropriate physical care. There has been a broad and growing consensus on these issues. Beyond that, there are differences between what Katz Rothman has called family-centred and feminist perspectives, and between advocates of 'natural' childbirth and advocates of choice (Katz Rothman 1982). However, these divisions can be overemphasized. In the 1990s we see a general alignment between advocates of natural birth and advocates of choice. This has come about because research evidence has consistently shown that interventions in childbirth confer risks or side-effects as well as benefits (when used appropriately). This has led to an understanding that 'unnecessary' intervention should be avoided. There is much scope for debate around what is necessary, but the principle of critically appraising the effectiveness of interventions has gained support. We also see a convergence of family-centred and feminist approaches. This can be attributed to the influence of feminism on mainstream beliefs. There is now a widespread agreement that women should have control over their body and be able to exercise choice. Several organizations representing a family-centred approach would now say that issues of gender inequality are central to maternity issues. On the whole there is considerably more agreement than dissent.

For example, the New Zealand Parents' Centre began and continues to be overtly family oriented. Dobbie (1990) described the early New Zealand Parents' Centre as advocating 'a more natural, more compassionate handling of the maternity scene . . . fostering better parent–child relationships and happier families'. At the same time she concluded of the women involved from the earliest days, 'Their feet were on the path of women's liberation, although they would not have thought of it like that at the time' (Dobbie 1990).

The childbirth movement has challenged the notion that development necessarily equals progress (Oakley 1984, Donnison 1988). In some respects, it has sought to rediscover traditional skills and values in new circumstances. This is true particularly of aspects of midwifery practice and care.

The movement has not observed passively. Those involved have created information and advocacy services to fill the gaps in statutory provision. They have also developed models of woman-centred care, including childbirth preparation classes, breastfeeding counselling, mother-to-mother support, special situations contact registers, and so on. Services to meet fathers' needs, though less well developed, have also been addressed. Antenatal classes for couples have been provided by the NCT for well over 20 years, and more recently by other organizations such as the Active Birth Movement. However, most successful of all the changes achieved for men has been the campaign for fathers to be 'allowed' to be present for the birth of their children, not least because this change in attitude has been fully adopted throughout the National Health Service (NHS). Indeed, so successful was the campaign that those men, or women, who do not feel comfortable about being together as a couple during birth sometimes feel they must assert themselves to be allowed to exercise choice. During 1994 most broadsheet newspapers discussed the topic. Through voluntary initiatives, such as those described, otherwise hidden needs have been revealed, and ways of meeting them have been developed and demonstrated to the statutory sector.

Oakley and Houd researched what they called the 'alternative perinatal services' in 10 countries (Canada, Denmark, France, former Federal Republic of Germany, The Netherlands, Sweden, USSR, UK, USA and former Yugoslavia) as part of a World Health Organization survey (WHO) (Oakley and Houd 1990, WHO 1985). Eight of the study countries were found to have user organizations contributing, in a broad sense, to perinatal care. The contributions made included both actual services to women or parents and lobbying to influence the range of services and quality of care provided by the official system.

Oakley and Houd found common concerns among the childbirth organizations studied. The concerns were the limitation of women's choice associated with developments in perinatal care; and lack of attention to pregnancy, birth and parenthood being a continuing process integral to 'the totality of human social life'. They found that the alternative services provided by user organizations emphasized the need to meet the individual needs of childbearing women, and the social significance of childbirth, as opposed to the idea of birth as a medical event. More specifically, they found that three themes were likely to be prominent in the history of maternity user organizations: insufficient choice of place of birth, poor conditions in hospital and overuse of medical procedures and technology in childbirth. The authors emphasized that no division was made by user organizations between the 'narrow health care needs and wider social needs of parents' (Oakley and Houd 1990).

The NCT, first established as the Natural Childbirth Association in 1956, was one of the very earliest maternity user organizations. However, on the other side of the world, in New Zealand, the Natural Childbirth Group began in the early 1950s, changing its name to the Parents' Centre in 1952. Both these organizations based their early activities on the teaching of Dr Grantly Dick-Read (1933, 1952). They promoted natural birth and were family oriented.

In the UK, another general interest maternity organization soon followed the NCT. The Association for Improvements in Maternity Services (AIMS) was founded in 1960 by Sally Willington, a woman motivated by her own experience. Willington wrote to a national newspaper about the inadequacies of her antenatal care and 'a deluge' of complaints from other women arrived (AIMS 1991). Known initially as the Society for the Prevention of Cruelty to Pregnant Women, AIMS was particularly oriented to meeting women's needs rather than the needs of families. It began campaigning for more hospital beds and a national epidural service, mirroring the concerns of pre-war women's organizations (Lewis 1990). However, by 1981 the emphasis had changed to 'the right of the mother to experience normal physiological childbirth without interference unless she wants it or there are clear indications that it is needed' (Beech 1981).

Oakley sees this switch by AIMS to 'the natural childbirth model' as evidence that 'the underlying conflict between users and providers of care was precisely centred on (the) dispute about the ideology and statistics of normality versus pathology' (Oakley 1984).

While Oakley is right to emphasize the change towards a natural childbirth perspective as a fundamental change for AIMS, the ideology underpinning their lobbying remained consistent: the ideology of choice for women. Interestingly as AIMS, along with other user organizations, has gained in confidence, the emphasis with which they advocate women's choice has increased. In the above quote from 1981, Beech indicates that there are two legitimate reasons for 'interference': the woman's choice and 'clear indications that it is needed' (Beech 1981). In the 1990s Beech would be unlikely to suggest that there might be reasons to override a woman's choice of care, for it is now widely recognized that there is no consensus about 'clear indications', nor about when (if ever) it is legitimate to act against the expressed wish of a conscious woman.

Also, in 1960, the International Childbirth Education Association (ICEA) was founded in the USA. The ICEA, like the NCT in England and Parents' Centres in New Zealand, was keen to promote natural childbirth techniques. However, the medicalized American birth environment made it quite impossible to relax, move freely and behave spontaneously. In *The American Way of Birth*, Jessica Mitford (1993) described the treatment routinely meted out to women in American hospitals in the 1950s and more recently. This involved women receiving a cocktail of narcotics, sedatives and other drugs, being made to lie flat on their back with legs raised, bent, wide apart and strapped into position; and being given an episiotomy and forceps.

The ICEA suggested there were 'two pillars of a happy birth – childbirth education and support during labour' (ICEA 1966). The education provided was influenced by the work of Grantly Dick-Read, but other methods of preparation for labour, particularly the Lamaze approach, were felt to be more suitable. The Dick-Read method was based on the woman being able to behave more or less as she wished, without interruptions. It required 'patient attendance during labour', a 'calm and peaceful atmosphere' and companionship (Allen 1990). Lamaze taught a psychoprophylactic, or conditioned response, approach to preparing for birth. This was found more effective as a means of pain control where interventions including the lithotomy position and stirrups were the norm. The emphasis of ICEA 'education' was more on adapting to the system than on changing the system: 'Women were taught to request politely that only leg and not hand restraints be used' (Katz Rothman 1982). 'Support during labour' was interpreted in a directive way; the idea of having a 'labour coach', and particularly a 'husband-coached labour' became fashionable: 'In ideal circumstances, the husband must be able to both *supervise* and support his wife during labour' (Sousa 1976, emphasis added).

The American Society for Psychoprophylactics in Obstetrics (ASPO) formed in 1960 was also 'geared specifically to hospital and the American way of birth' (Katz Rothman 1982). Unlike the European organizations Oakley and Houd describe, ASPO was uncritical of medicalized childbirth. The 1961 training course said:

> In all cases the woman should be encouraged to respect her doctor's word as final. . . . It is most important to stress that her job and his are completely separate. He is responsible for her physical well-being and that of her baby. She is responsible for controlling herself and her behaviour.
>
> (Katz Rothman 1982)

As time passed, the ICEA and other American maternity organizations began to question seriously the prevailing medical system of care. The National Association of Parents and Professionals for Safe Alternatives in Childbirth (NAPSAC), established in 1976, brought together groups, including lay midwives, who had reason to challenge the *status quo* in American obstetrics. They advocated a more family-friendly, woman-centred approach. Nancy Mills, a midwife who learned to practise by attending births as a friend rather than through formal hospital-based teaching, explained at a NAPSAC conference what she saw as her role at a birth:

> I see myself as going in and being a helper, being an attendant. Sometimes it means I sit near the room. Sometimes I play with the kids or I do some cooking. Sometimes I sit with the woman. Sometimes I help a husband assist the woman. Some families need more help than others but it's easy to go in and see how you can fit in and see where you are needed and how you can fill that role. . . . I know it helps when I say to a woman, 'I know how you feel. I know its harder than you thought it was going to be, but you can do it.' It is a very important thing that women are not left alone in labour.
>
> (Stewart and Stewart 1976)

The values and concerns expressed in this excerpt are consistent with the themes Oakley and Houd (1990) suggested were likely to be prominent in the history of maternity organizations. Implicit is the belief that the place of birth should not be restricted to hospital, that conditions for birth should be designed not to disturb the family's prefered behaviour, and that social and emotional means of support should be used before considering medical procedures. *Spiritual Midwifery* (Gaskin 1975), published by lay midwives in the USA and imported to Britain, epitomised these values and inspired campaigners.

Maternity organizations similar to NAPSAC exist in other countries. For instance, Parents and Childbirth founded in Denmark in 1970 has had an important role to play in humanizing the perinatal services (Houd 1988). Although there has been a strong tradition of midwifery in that country, important changes have affected the quality of maternity care. During the 1960s and 1970s births moved from home into hospital and in 1973 a centralized system of employing midwives was introduced, disrupting continuity of local midwifery care. At the same time a routine system of risk scoring was introduced. After successful lobbying, perinatal guidelines published in 1985 had dropped all reference to risk groups. Instead, there was evidence of a woman-centred approach, 'The perinatal period is a normal period of a family's life. The woman, her family and close friends should be central. The midwife, doctors and other staff are only there to support the woman and her family' (Houd 1988).

As well as these general interest maternity organizations, dozens of specific interest groups have been formed relating to birth, breastfeeding and parenting (Durward and Evans 1990). A few, like the Active Birth Movement and the Society to Support Home Confinement, fit the Oakley and Houd criteria of being concerned about place of birth, conditions in hospital and use of medical procedures and technology. Others focus their attention elsewhere but share a basic concern to provide parents with good information and emotional support.

The WHO investigation *Having a Baby in Europe* found that user organizations were often formed on the basis of someone's personal experience and functions often included providing information on birth issues, producing leaflets or a newsletter, facilitating an exchange of views between parents and health professionals, gathering information on maternity services, collecting experiences and attitudes of parents, antenatal education classes/discussion, practical help with formal complaints about services, fund-raising, organizing seminars or conferences, representing the interests of childbearing women and their partners to the media and to government, and lobbying and organizing campaigns (WHO 1985).

Maternity user's organizations in the UK include SANDS (Stillbirth and Neonatal Death Society), SATFA (Support Around Termination for Fetal Abnormality), MAMA (Meet a Mum Association), and the Association of Breastfeeding Mothers. Within the NCT, special interest groups have grown up – including the Breastfeeding Promotion Group, ParentAbility and working mothers' groups – and have developed a distinct identity of their own. The Working Mothers' Association grew out of the Clapham NCT working mothers' group and was recently relaunched as Parents at Work. Locally, there are innumerable support groups taking an interest in maternity issues; one such is the Sheffield Black Women's Group.

The WHO study group questioned why alternative perinatal services develop and put forward three hypotheses, namely that alternative perinatal services are most likely to develop in areas (a) where the official services emphasize clinical (medical/technological) care rather than social needs and where care takes place nearly exclusively in hospital; (b) where there is an absence of continuity of care, from the same person or a small team of individuals; and (c) where the position and status of midwives *vis-à-vis* obstetricians is threatened. They concluded that these hypotheses were confirmed by the data collected (WHO 1985).

With these ideas in mind, it is easier to see what it is that unites and separates the organizations set up to support and represent childbearing women and their families in the UK.

MATERNITY GROUPS IN THE UK

There are currently three sizeable, general interest organizations providing services and lobbying around maternity issues in the UK: the NCT, AIMS and the Maternity Alliance. NCT now has approximately 50,000 members and 380 branches throughout England, Wales, Scotland and Northern Ireland. It has one office in London with 25 staff. AIMS has up to 1000 members at any time, depending on the level of interest in lobbying for change in maternity care. It is run entirely by volunteers. Maternity Alliance is an umbrella organization uniting parent groups, user organizations, trade unions, health bodies, and others with an interest. It has seven paid staff.

Maternity Alliance was founded in 1980. Its objectives were different from those of both the NCT and AIMS in that, rather than focusing specifically on childbirth or maternity services, Maternity Alliance has focused on the social context of birth. Much of their work concerns employment rights, maternity and child benefit, the effects of poverty and other forms of inequality. Now, in the 1990s, they employ a lawyer working on sex discrimination and maternity rights; they have an active Black and Minority Ethnic Working Group and a Disability Awareness Working Group. They have led or been closely associated with many campaigns including Maternity Emergency, focusing on the erosion of mothers' benefits and employment rights, and the Save Child Benefit Campaign. They promoted the first parliamentary bill to establish a statutory right to paternity leave and have campaigned for 18 weeks maternity leave as a minimum. Most recently, they have lobbied the government on the implementation of the EC directive on the protection of pregnant women at work.

Other work has included publications for health professionals on helping women write a birth plan; a postnatal pack, *New Lives*, for community groups to use; and a resource pack on support services for very young mothers. In 1993 they held the first ever residential conference for parents with a disability and have since launched a charter and survey report (Goodman 1994). Though they have such a broad brief, Maternity Alliance has been no less concerned about birth issues. In 1989 they drew attention to the increase in Caesarean sections and other interventions in labour (Maternity Alliance 1989).

AIMS describes itself as a pressure group. As the name states clearly, it has a mission to change the maternity services. AIMS' strategies have been characterized by a direct, sometimes confrontational, approach and its members have not balked at criticizing practices they believed to be wrong. The organization works directly with women, advising them on their rights, and taking up individual cases where some injustice has apparently been done. Unlike the NCT, which has put most of its resources into training antenatal teachers and breast-feeding counsellors, and developing a nationwide network of branches offering social support, AIMS has remained a smaller organization with a less diverse brief. Its energies and resources have been channelled into publishing information and policy documents and campaigning for change.

AIMS is inspired more by feminist values than family-centredness. It seeks to highlight both the benefits of 'natural' birth and to advocate choice. To AIMS the quality of the maternity services is one of the most important women's issues. One AIMS member, Sandar Warshal, explained that to them the main issues at stake are women's rights, rather than the quality of the experience of giving birth *per se*. In her terms, 'AIMS members are not what you would describe as "birthy women".'

In contrast with AIMS, the NCT, pioneers of antenatal classes for couples, aims to address the needs of parents. As an organization the NCT has distanced itself from feminism. Public references to the male-domination of obstetrics were consciously avoided as recently as 1986 (Kitzinger 1990). More recently, the NCT's evidence to the Health Select Committee introduced gender as an important issue in maternity care (Health Select Committee 1992). It is noteworthy that while many of the services provided are aimed at meeting the needs of families, the overwhelming majority of NCT members and office-holders are women, and training to become an NCT antenatal teacher or breastfeeding counsellor is open to women only. So, in important respects the NCT is very much a women's organization.

Despite their rather different concerns and objectives, NCT, AIMS and Maternity Alliance share the view that the role of midwives is central to providing woman-centred maternity services. The following section looks in more detail at the policies and strategies of the NCT. In particular, it considers when and how the position and status of midwives was identified as important for childbearing women.

NCT POLICY AND STRATEGIES

The primary aim of those who founded the Natural Childbirth Association (NCA) was 'to enable women to experience childbirth without fear'. Members of the organization set about providing women with information and 'training' for birth. They aimed to reduce the amount of drugs needed in a normal labour and to help women avoid routine episiotomy. Their approach to preparing women for giving birth was inspired and directed by the NCA's first president, Grantly Dick-Read, best known for his book *Childbirth without Fear* (1952).

Influenced by their own experiences, the founding members also had a personal commitment to helping other women. Although the word 'empowering' would not have been used then, the women involved wanted to give others the best possible chance of a good birth experience. They wanted to see an end to fear and pain and a sense of loss. They knew birth could enrich women's lives, leaving a lasting sense of fulfilment. The style of the NCA during the first few years could perhaps be summed up as radical enthusiasm.

By 1961, the organization had obtained charitable status, and changed its name to The National Childbirth Trust (NCT). In that year it appointed an obstetrician, Stanley Perchard, as chairman and consciously set about presenting a more conciliatory, orthodox face to the world (Kitzinger 1990). In particular, the NCT was anxious not to antagonize health professionals. This meant avoiding challenging their authority, knowledge or control.

Perchard produced notes on 'Medical and professional etiquette and the NCT'. They read, 'The best interest of the mother demands that she has every confidence in those who have the clinical responsibility for her safety and that of her baby. The ultimate aim of the Trust should be to interest the doctors and midwives so that they actively participate in the mother's training, or *better still take charge of it*. Where this is not possible the training should *at all costs* avoid dividing the mother's loyalty or impairing her confidence in her professional attendants' (NCT 1966, emphasis added).

The NCT had published its first leaflets about the process of birth (NCT 1960), exercises and posture during pregnancy (NCT 1962), breathing control in labour (NCT 1964a), and breastfeeding and caring for the new baby (NCT 1964b). It encouraged parents to believe that 'labour is a job of work for which most healthy women are well equipped'. Despite on the one hand promoting the idea of childbirth as a normal physiological process, on the other, the NCT was anxious not to challenge health professionals too openly. They attempted to get round this potential contradiction by instructing the women who came to classes to behave with tact and charm, by suggesting to doctors that women who had been to classes would be more compliant patients, and by appealing to doctors' paternalism to indulge women at a vulnerable time in their lives (Kitzinger 1990). At this stage midwives were not identified as a distinct group, separate from doctors (Kitzinger 1990). This is perhaps not surprising as the midwives practising in hospital were already well incorporated into the 'obstetric team' (Donnison 1988).

Originally, teachers sent 'consent forms' to GPs informing them that their patient had enlisted for a course of antenatal preparation and asking for consent. By 1969 this had become a 'letter of notification' stating that classes would include education in the process of labour, and in the practice of relaxation and breathing techniques for use during labour. The letter made clear that obstetric advice would not be offered and women would be asked to take any questions about their own physical care to their GP.

In the early 1960s the NCT approach to birth preparation moved away from Dick-Read's teaching towards the Lamaze approach (Kitzinger 1990). The *Helpers' Handbook* for 1966 said, 'There is no "best" method and it is important to emphasize whenever an opportunity arises that the NCT is in no way tied to any one method of preparation for childbirth. ... New ideas and theories evolve, new techniques develop. Not one of our HQ teachers would say that they are teaching now in exactly the same way that they taught even a year ago' (NCT 1966). It stated that the NCT was *not* saying that training for childbirth would mean *effortless* childbirth, but that it was hoped preparation would 'reduce pain-consciousness'. The NCT did *not* believe women should be denied the use of drugs and analgesics if they felt the need of them (NCT 1966).

The NCT support for breastfeeding was a natural follow-through from the wish to humanize the birth experience. To facilitate breastfeeding the NCT advocated rooming-in and demand-feeding. In 1967 a separate committee, the Breastfeeding Promotion Group, was formed, taking responsibility for NCT publications on breastfeeding, such as the leaflet *Why Breastfeed?* (NCT 1968a), and for the training and registration of breastfeeding counsellors.

Over the years, NCT branches developed a tradition of disseminating ideas about good practice in maternity care by organizing study days for members and for health professionals. As midwives were required to attend study days as part of their on-going training, the NCT could attract them with interesting speakers and a local venue. This was acknowledged by the President of the Royal College of Midwives when she addressed an ICEA convention. She explained that, 'A practising midwife (in Britain) must take a refresher course every five years ... Many seminars are arranged by the National Childbirth Trust and a considerable number of members attend these.... Many of them speak of the great benefit gained by such attendance' (ICEA 1966).

Although some midwives and physiotherapists also attended NCT classes to observe, there was considerable suspicion and resentment of the NCT among midwives during the 1960s and the early 1970s. There was certainly no sense at that time that the NCT and midwives shared common objectives. The NCT Journal (Spring 1978) quoted from an exchange of correspondence in the *Nursing Times*. One midwife had written, 'Midwives should be aware that our previous autonomy and autocracy may well be eroded by the current trend of lay folk teaching the professionals how to teach' (*Nursing Times*, 10 November 1977). But someone responded, 'Until "professionals" begin seriously to involve clients in planning their own care it is inevitable, though not undesirable, that such organizations as the NCT will exist. What we should remember is that the majority of members of this and similar organizations are middle-class women who are able to vocalize their needs. Working-class women's needs are similarly, if not more, neglected' (*Nursing Times*, 1 December 1977). However, a third correspondent asked, 'Does this mean that our expensive statutory training and costly service provisions do not enable us to meet the real needs of those we are employed and paid to care for?' (*Nursing Times*, 12 January 1978). She went on to say that professionals were being 'elbowed out of the way by well-meaning amateurs'.

The NCT was conscious of its image and tried to avoid reinforcing negative impressions. The 1966 *Helpers Handbook* had a section on 'pitfalls to avoid', described as notes designed 'to avoid mistakes that have occasionally been made in the past'. The notes included, 'Please avoid giving the impression that you think you "know it all" because you have had a baby (or two) and "it worked", or because you have attended a seminar – or sat with mothers in labour. Please avoid expressing dogmatic opinions on matters of medical technique. Please avoid criticising those who attended mothers antenatally and in labour' (NCT 1966).

Despite efforts to play down conflict, NCT members and those who had been to NCT classes were unable to throw off a negative reputation among midwives. The label 'NCT-type' was used pejoratively. While the term is still referred to (Green *et al.* 1988), gradually over the 1970s and 1980s the attitudes of many midwives changed.

Historical context

To understand the situation of midwives and the NCT better, it may help to consider them in historical context. The NCT grew into a nationwide network at a time when there was a revolution in childbirth taking place. There were more maternity beds in hospitals, and many more babies being born away from home. In 1937, 25% of births took place in hospital. By 1954, two years before the NCA was founded, the proportion had increased substantially to 64%. However, the fastest growth in hospital delivery took place between 1963 and

1972 when the rate leapt from 68% to 91% (Oakley 1984). By 1987, less than 1% of births were at home.

Despite there being no evidence on which to base assertions of the benefits of universal hospital confinement (Campbell and MacFarlane 1987), specialist doctors were confident about, and persuasive in promoting, their contribution to maternal and perinatal health. The opening chapter of a medical book on the maternity services entitled 'Progress in the 1960s and problems for the 1970s', argued that '. . . a concerted effort on behalf of the medical profession, as a whole, could achieve a very much higher proportion of hospital confinements' (Smith 1970). The author concluded, 'The considerable variation in perinatal mortality within Britain *must be* mainly due to variations in the quality of medical care available to fetuses. Just as we have a responsibility to a postnatal child even when parental attitudes are not cooperative, so we must increasingly assume similar responsibilities in respect of the fetus (Smith 1970, emphasis added).

However, another chapter in the same volume reported an 'absence of any clear relation between rate of hospital confinement and perinatal mortality'. The authors concluded:

> *When the future of the maternity services in this country is considered, the main object must be to ensure that the best possible use is made of resources and that any new developments should be in areas in which the potential gains are greatest. On the evidence of recent experience it is by no means certain that the trend towards increasing hospital confinement apparent since 1963 is the best policy.*
>
> (Ashford and Fryer 1970)

Without clear evidence, the claim of obstetricians that medicine, the use of technology and hospitalization would reduce mortality and morbidity and improve the quality of life was widely accepted. Both politicians and the public were persuaded. Successive government reports – the Cranbrook Report (1959), the Peel Report (1970) and the Short Report (1980) – have advocated confinement in hospital (Oakley 1984). The importance of medicine in maternity care was promoted at all levels, so that reference could be made to 'doctor's orders' without any hint of irony, as in this example:

> *. . . (the older mother) may have to watch her health more carefully, obey her doctor's orders and attend antenatal check-ups even more conscientiously than a younger one.*
>
> (*Good Housekeeping* 1961)

As hospital beds became more widely available during the 1940s and 1950s it was seen by many women as a bonus to be offered one. Middle-class women, who had better facilities at home, were sometimes envious of less privileged women who were offered a hospital bed (Lewis 1990). However, women's experiences of birth in hospital were less widely discussed than the belief that hospital birth was modern and safe. From its earliest years, the NCT had evidence that women who went into hospital often felt isolated and vulnerable. The surroundings and the staff were unfamiliar and the atmosphere very different from home.

Hospitals were hierarchical with doctors at the top and patients at the bottom of the pyramid. Midwifery practice was bound by inflexible rules. Midwives were required to 'manage' women so that they behaved as the regime expected them to. Women's labour reports, published in local NCT newsletters during the 1960s, show that those women who gave birth at home referred to their 'midwife', while those who had their baby in hospital talked about the 'nurse' or 'sister'.

The 1968 Annual Report quoted a letter from an NCT teacher who was also a midwife which outlined some of the obstacles to more woman–centred care. She said in her hospital there was 'no time to talk to the patients (sic) and remind them what to do (during labour); still the old feeling that the patient is best kept in ignorance; and absolutely no comprehension of what the patient might be feeling'. She went on 'I really wish it were possible for all midwives to have babies before completing their training, perhaps then they could have a little more compassion'(NCT 1968b).

This view reflected a belief that mothers could and would identify with and support other mothers. It was felt that much that was wrong with maternity care was the result of doctors and midwives cutting themselves off emotionally from the processes of birth and breastfeeding as women experienced them. It was felt that having a baby oneself would wake health professionals up to the pain and potential pleasures of having a baby. As a principle, women were only eligible to train as an NCT antenatal teacher if they had given birth. This could be either a vaginal or a Caesarean birth because it was felt that the emotional feelings were the important thing, rather than the physical. Similarly, women were only eligible to train as an NCT breastfeeding counsellor if they had breastfed a baby. For this training it was considered important to have established and maintained breastfeeding, overcoming any problems experienced. Thus, a minimum period of lactation was specified.

Medical control

During the first half of the twentieth century, working–class and middle-class women in the UK were anxious for more medical care, greater access to hospital beds and more pain relief (Roberts 1984, Lewis 1990). However, in seeking solutions to their need for privacy, rest, comfort and safety in childbirth, women also lost control. Birth came to be viewed as a medical event rather than a normal life-event (Lewis 1990). Obstetricians took control of childbirth away not only from mothers but also from midwives and GPs (Oakley 1984, Donnison 1988). The primary objective of obstetricians has been to reduce perinatal and maternal mortality. Their methods of achieving this have been questioned (Tew 1977, Donnison 1988, Oakley and Houd 1990, Wagner 1994) and they have been criticized for ignoring the significance of morbidity in mothers and babies, particularly as mortality rates have fallen. In particular, obstetricians have tended to overlook the needs of women and their role as producers of healthy babies and providers of care for themselves and for their babies. Rather than seeing women as active users of the maternity services and participants in decision-making, the medical model of maternity care has cast women as passive and rather unreliable.

Gordon Bourne, a well-known obstetrician, addressed an NCT conference in the early 1970s on the active management of labour. The report of his presentation read:

> *If the sick child is safest delivered by a carefully timed labour, surely this is good enough for the well child too. . . . What is good enough for the abnormal is good enough for the normal. . . . In unassisted labour you have a baby over which you have no control, and a uterus over which you have no control. . . . I am prepared to accept that loss (of biological rhythm) in return for safety.*
>
> (NCT 1974a)

This illustrates the way obstetricians have tended to see themselves as saving vulnerable babies from a hostile environment. The NCT questioned the use of medical interventions. In particular, the use of procedures designed for coping with complications of labour being used when the labour was proceeding normally. For example, the explicit policy in one hospital was that all women should be given an episiotomy so that no-one in need would be missed. In contrast, older midwives would recall taking pride in the number of women they cared for who gave birth without a cut or a tear.

The same routine, inflexible approach was evident in other aspects of 'management'. In pregnancy, it became the vogue to monitor weight gain closely. Those who put on 'too much' were literally 'told off'. During labour women were given an enema, shaved, bathed and confined to bed without access to food or drink. After the birth, breastfeeding was restricted and controlled down to the finest detail.

The services failed to take account of women's needs. It was normal for women to wait for hours in clinics because antenatal appointments were booked in blocks (Oakley 1984). Women saw different staff on each visit to hospital, leading to repetition and duplication. Though pregnant women know their body intimately and continuously, their knowledge was not valued. Often, the same tests and assessments would be done by the GP, the midwife and the hospital doctor (Oakley 1984). Advice was often conflicting. It was easy for health professionals to be patronizing to women they did not know as individuals. The short exchanges that were possible as women were conveyed from weeing to weighing to blood pressure checks and to palpation and, perhaps, an internal examination were often empty and meaningless.

Within the NCT there was discussion about good practice – where it occurred – as well as concern about bad practice. Knowledge of positive examples of care inspired NCT members to work towards improving care in their local areas. In antenatal classes, teachers discussed with parents how to go about getting what they wanted. They learned from each other to write down their questions in advance, so as not to be put off by the consultant. As much as possible, women made a practice of avoiding having discussions with the doctor while still lying down and semi-naked. They took someone with them to antenatal appointments and to hospital in labour for moral support. Increasingly, they found out about alternatives and stated their preferences.

However, the approach of giving information and teaching skills to a small minority of women who came to NCT classes did not solve the problems of getting improvements for *all* women.

Initiatives of the 1970s

The NCT became more politicized during the 1970s. It began to value women's experiences more openly. As the NCT network developed, the organization was directly in touch with the experiences of thousands of women. As they talked to each other at meetings and through the newsletters, and as antenatal teachers and breastfeeding counsellors compared notes, particular patterns emerged.

Increasingly, links were made with individuals from a range of disciplines who questioned the way maternity care was moving. Multidisciplinary meetings were held to discuss policies and publish new ideas. A group of respected people were invited to become formal advisers. Research evidence became a central part of the debate about appropriate care. The Royal College of Obstetricians and Gynaecologists (RCOG) was lobbied but obstetricians were no longer invited to chair the executive committee. By the end of the decade, the NCT began to look to midwives as the group potentially able to provide supportive, responsive care.

Dissenting professionals, like the South American obstetrician Caldeyro-Barcia, who wrote about 'humanized management of normal labour'(1979) and the Dutch obstetrician, Professor G. J. Kloosterman, inspired courage and dissent. Kloosterman said:

> *It is the duty of the obstetrician to protect the large number of completely healthy pregnant women against unnecessary interference, impatience, over-estimation of one's capacities and human meddlesomeness.*

> (NCT 1974a)

Increasing numbers of women were looking for attendants who had confidence in them and in the normality of the birth process. As well as the NCT, they joined groups such as AIMS, the Society to Support Home Confinements and, later, the Active Birth Movement.

Changing awareness

The tone of the NCT's 1974 Annual Report was not very different from the tone of the leaflets for parents produced in the 1960s. It referred to NCT antenatal classes as 'aiming to lead women to know what to expect at the time of childbirth and how to work with their own bodies, adapt to different experiences and *co-operate with their attendants*' (NCT 1974b, emphasis added).

However, by the end of the decade there was a more challenging debate under way. In 1979, in the NCT's *Teachers' Broadsheet*, a teacher asked, 'Should I be preparing parents for a strong possibility of an induction and an almost certain episiotomy? Should parents just accept it?' (NCT 1979a). Sheila Kitzinger, herself an active NCT teacher and teacher tutor as well as an anthropologist and author of books for women, responded:

> *It is not enough to be teachers who simply reassure women and prepare them to accept whatever happens in hospitals. . . . When we see our role only as teaching women to accept the 'inevitable' and making them feel comfortable about it we are actually supporting present-day obstetric practices and helping to block the spontaneous protest which would otherwise come from many women who don't know why they are having their labours accelerated or their membranes artificially ruptured, their perineal hair shaved or suppositories given.*

> (NCT 1979a)

Health professionals

It became clear that the NCT could further its objective of ensuring that childbirth was a positive experience for women and their partners by lobbying health professionals to change their attitudes and resist rigid labour ward protocols. Philippa Micklethwait, President of the NCT, addressed a study group of the RCOG on parents' needs, suggesting that lessons could be learned from the labour reports received by NCT antenatal teachers about factors that women found helped reduce distress and raise their pain threshold. She referred to midwives and doctors who were kind, encouraging and interested in the 'patient' as a person, and staff who were very good at explaining what they were doing. She praised those who discussed the situation and obtained the mother's informed consent before giving injections or setting up drips; and those who – although for them it may be just another birth in a busy week – could nevertheless sense the excitement and the feeling of a uniquely important event for this particular mother and father.

Philippa Micklethwait also established a rights of parents discussion group, with representatives drawn from education, general practice, midwifery, obstetrics, physiotherapy and social science. In 1977 the group published a list of 10 standards of care, 'Expectations of a pregnant woman in relation to her treatment', which might be seen as an early pregnant women's charter. The list included the need for factual information, an assumption that labour would start normally unless there was a medical reason for induction, that labour would proceed normally without intervention unless there were indications that this might be unsafe, that alternative methods of pain relief would be explained during pregnancy and that choices could be made in labour without pressure.

The list went on that induction or acceleration of labour should be discussed before a decision was taken, that women should have a labour companion if they wished, and 'if it were possible' women should have someone around during labour who had given some antenatal care. After the birth, the mother should be able to hold the baby as soon as possible and spend some time holding and feeding, if she wished and there were no medical problems. She should not be separated from her baby 'unless it was essential' and be allowed to feed the baby at any time. Finally, professional advice and support would should continue for as long as it was needed.

The conclusions were published in the *Midwives Chronicle*, the *Midwife & Health Visitor*, the *Nursing Times* and the *British Medical Journal* (Mickelthwait *et al.* 1978). By facilitating this group and targeting the midwifery and medical press, the NCT was deliberately creating ways of initiating dialogue and presenting positive models of care to doctors and midwives.

Research

Research has played a crucial role in the growing strength of the childbirth movement and in the influence of the NCT. In the early days, Grantly Dick-Read had been dismissive of the need for research, believing that he already knew what it was important to know (Sheila Kitzinger, personal communication). He believed labour could be understood in terms of Divine purpose (Dick-Read 1933). His closest followers have taken the same view. For example, on pain in labour, Briance, founder of the Natural Childbirth Association, said:

> *Dr Dick-Read proved to his own satisfaction that the Creator certainly did not create pain for women in childbirth* because there is no mechanism for pain in normal labour. *The pain of labour is a man projected distortion of the true picture of natural birth, a misconception.*
>
> (Briance 1982, emphasis in original)

Without systematic and appropriate evidence it is difficult to establish what is unsubstantiated prejudice and what is reliable knowledge. Many people believe their own perspective is important and that others are wrong or their understandings are irrelevant. The merits of competing claims can only be assessed by rigorous research. Obstetricians have tended to believe that medical training and attendance at numerous deliveries provides a more important understanding of birth than a woman's personal experience. They have tended to dismiss women's views, particularly if expressed with emotion. The medical model of maternity care led to the assumption that little could be gained from listening to women.

Sheila Kitzinger did much to change that view. By writing about women's experiences she opened up a wealth of knowledge (1962, 1978, 1979a,b). Anyone reading her books realized that giving birth was a profound experience for women and becoming a parent moved both mothers and fathers to the core. As well as highlighting the emotional significance of birth by asking parents what they went through and how they felt, she found out about women's experiences of procedures such as episiotomy (Kitzinger and Walters 1981) and epidural (Kitzinger 1987). She conducted descriptive studies, published by the NCT, which showed in detail the physical and emotional outcomes associated with these interventions. Later, the NCT went on to survey women's experiences of postnatal infections (Greenshields 1988), rupture of the membranes in labour (Borton *et al.* 1989), perineal care and trauma (Greenshields and Hulme 1993), and the maternity services (NCT 1992, Newburn 1993).

Prior to the 1970s the NCT, like midwifery practice and much of obstetrics, was not research oriented. Looking back, Sheila Kitzinger said of the early

NCT, 'We were not research oriented in any way. We were making assumptions. I started (the NCT research work) with tremendous opposition. We were into comfort not confusion. You concentrated on clear instructions and didn't get bogged down' (personal communication, 1994).

There were notable exceptions. Constance Benyon, obstetrician and chair of the NCT Executive Committee in 1962, was one example. She conducted research comparing women allowed to behave instinctively during the second stage of labour with those given formal pushing instructions. She concluded that there was no difference in the duration of the second stage (Benyon 1957). While this work is found valuable today (Watson 1994) it was not granted much attention at the time. Crucially, much of clinical practice was not research based, and was not reviewed in the light of new research evidence.

The more women and professionals began using, reviewing and doing relevant research themselves, the more assumptions were shaken. Doris Haire's polemical but firmly grounded, *The Cultural Warping of Childbirth* (1972), was very influential. She went on to unearth information on the effects of diagnostic ultrasound (Haire 1984). Marjorie Tew, a statistician, made a crucial contribution to the childbirth debate accidentally when she discovered that the mortality rates for home births looked very favourable next to those for hospital births (Tew 1977). She was invited by the NCT to join a group including Iain Chalmers, Martin Richards, G. J. Kloosterman, Luke Zander and Cloe Fisher to take part in a series of meetings 'about the direction that modern obstetrics appeared to be taking under the impetus of advances in technology and the increasing bureaucracy involved with medical care'. A collection of papers was published as *The Place of Birth* (Kitzinger and Davis 1978).

In addition to evidence on the place of birth, attention was directed towards the evidence on particular procedures in common use. Mona Romney, a midwife, conducted trials on the use of enemas (Romney and Gordon 1981) and perineal shaving (Romney 1980). AIMS members, who seemed to thrive on crossing swords with health professionals, began asking on what evidence they were justifying interventions. 'Around about 1976, we began to scrutinize the medical literature. We stopped saying "We don't like it". We started saying "Why are you doing it?" ' (Beverley Beech, AIMS, personal communication 1994).

In 1970 the NCT became involved in conducting a survey of users. A new maternity unit was proposed in Bath and the local branch of the NCT were provided with a one-in-ten sample of mothers to find out about the facilities they would like. The fact that this was *not* a survey of NCT members, but a representative sample of the childbearing population of Bath, provided useful evidence when the NCT was later challenged about whether it could speak for women generally. Among other things the survey showed that women had a preference for antenatal care from a GP rather than a hospital clinic (Dawson *et al.* 1971). It meant that they received continuity of care from the familiar family doctor, who was more easily accessible and whose waiting times were shorter. Women found the hospital clinics were less friendly, they saw different staff at each visit, often had transport problems, long waits and suffered from lack of privacy.

The women wanted more information on a wide range of subjects, believing generally that the more they knew the better. The vast majority said the most important matter for them in labour was having someone with them the whole time. Some women who had been persuaded to have their babies in hospital because it was considered to be safer were disillusioned when they found that they lost all privacy and received less attention than if they had stayed at home. Many said they would welcome less medical examination and more moral support from staff. Mothers felt strongly that they should be able to make their own choice about feeding their baby. Those who bottle-fed had felt an air of disapproval, yet those who breastfed felt they had received little encouragement and some reported that staff had bottle-fed the babies during the night (Dawson *et al.* 1971).

Women took back power by investigating the issues that mattered to them. When Sheila Kitzinger was gathering information for *The Good Birth Guide* (1979c), almost 2000 women wrote to her. The guide used a star rating system, in which hospitals were awarded a star if five women or more reported having been very happy with their experience. The guide stirred things up a lot, and people became angry when their local hospital did badly. It raised awareness among parents about what to look for in a hospital when trying to find one that would suit them. It also helped midwives who were trying to find a hospital where they could practise in the way they wished (Sheila Kitzinger, personal communication 1994). The book sold well and was later updated (Kitzinger 1983a).

Maternity care also received a lot of publicity when it became the subject of an inquiry by the popular television programme *That's Life*. The survey, involving 6000 respondents, highlighted how ordinary women of all social backgrounds want to make choices and receive sensitive care (Boyd and Sellers 1982). The authors of the *That's Life* study concluded that '... a good midwife is perhaps the single most important factor in determining whether a birth is enjoyed or not' (Boyd and Sellers 1982).

Induction

During the 1970s the aspect of care causing most concern was induction of labour. In December 1974 a letter from the NCT was published in a national newspaper saying that in some areas women were being asked to go into hospital a fortnight before Christmas, to have labour induced for professionals' convenience. The letter named no hospitals, but ended with the phrase 'No room at the inn?'. It resulted in the NCT receiving over a hundred requests for press interviews. Local reporters wanted to know whether this was happening in their area.

The following year the Department of Health and Social Security (DHSS) held an initial enquiry into the use of induction. At the time over a third of births in the UK were induced, the rate being much higher in some hospitals. In at least one hospital the only exceptions were women who arrived at hospital in established labour (personal communication 1975).

The NCT published a report on *Some Mothers' Experiences of Induced Labour* (Kitzinger 1975). Audrey Wise MP invited the NCT to present its findings and recommendations to an inter-party meeting at the House of Commons (December 1975). The NCT called for wide publication of the DHSS findings and conclusions so that ordinary people could be informed about what was going on and would have the opportunity to take part in the debate.

The NCT report on induction concluded that 'technical equipment' should be reserved for at-risk mothers who would benefit, that there should be sufficient staff available to provide women with support in labour, and that providing continuity of care should be a funding priority. It recommended that women should be able to give feedback to obstetricians and midwives about their policies. 'We urge the setting up of a study group consisting of hospital obstetricians, GP obstetricians, midwives and mothers to discover what the experience of labour means for women and to explore ways in which it can be improved' (Kitzinger 1975). The report also concluded that, 'Ultimately our culture of childbirth poses not only medical questions but ethical ones, and the way we have our babies is an expression of human values in our society for which (we all) are responsible' (Kitzinger 1975).

Government enquiries

During the 1970s there were numerous opportunities to put forward evidence to government investigating committees and respond to reports. The NCT sent evidence to the Committee on Voluntary Organizations in 1975 expressing the view that the healthy and normal aspects of childbirth were too often ignored 'in any medical list of statutory priorities'. The NCT felt more emphasis should be placed on the women's 'emotional wellbeing . . . and the family relationships'.

In 1980 the Short Report from the Parliamentary Social Services Committee on Perinatal and Neonatal Mortality came in for considerable criticism from the NCT, who said:

> *Care must be taken that over-zealous concern for the minority for whom very real problems exist, does not spill over to harm the majority, for whom birth is a normal and not a pathological process.*

> *Much better and more rigorous assessment of the effects of new technology (are needed), comparable to the attention given to new drugs.*

> *It is unethical to subject women to forms of intervention and treatment which have not been validated by properly controlled trials.*

(NCT 1980)

Midwives

The NCT had long been aware that the role of the midwife was central to the woman's experience of birth. What was not possible in the early days was to see midwives as a group as allies. Many, particularly hospital midwives, were seen as part of the opposition, as representing the system, even 'the enemy'.

During the 1970s and 1980s midwives' attitudes began to change. Gradually more married women were staying in employment and those who had a baby themselves were often profoundly affected by the experience. More independent thinkers were attracted to train as midwives, women who became involved in research (Kirkham 1989), in policy development (Page 1988) and informing women (Inch 1982). Some midwives who became well-known opinion leaders trained after qualifying as NCT antenatal teachers, for example Caroline Flint, Nicky Leap and Jean Davies. Penelope Samuel, midwife at the Bournemouth Midwife Unit, was formerly an NCT breastfeeding counsellor and chair of the NCT's Breastfeeding Promotion Group. They have often attributed aspects of their approach to midwifery to their experience of working with women within the NCT.

In 1976 two student midwives, Judy Rogers and Marianne Scruggs, who objected to the common practice in their hospital of inducing women on their 'expected date of delivery' decided to meet together regularly for mutual support. They went public about their concerns in a letter to *The Times*. They and the midwives who joined them became the Association of Radical Midwives (ARM), a support group for midwives concerned that the traditional skills of midwifery should not be lost (ARM 1986).

The NCT played an important part in helping to get ARM established by hosting a series of meetings to which about 40 women – midwives and members of ARM and AIMS – were invited to discuss the crucial situation in midwifery. The discussion covered the most obvious changes that had sprung from the increased number of births in hospital and routine interventions affecting all women. When births were in hospital there was more control by obstetricians although the labour was conducted by the midwife. It was suggested that 'Midwives are not encouraged to protest on behalf of their patients. Possibly the time has come for parents in their role as a consumer group to look at the difficulties facing midwives (NCT 1978).

The NCT was becoming increasingly conscious of the particular role of midwives and the need for its members to understand the difficulties midwives faced. The report of the NCT working party on antenatal care objected that midwives seemed to have vanished from clinics, to be replaced by nurses. It said:

The midwife is the expert on normal pregnancy and childbirth and it is she who must in the future be the central person in maternity care. The future of obstetrics in Britain depends on her. A good midwife does a great deal more than merely supervise a pregnancy and check that all is normal; she gives active caring and answers a woman's need for her pregnancy to be acknowledged as important, not simply in the physical sense, but because she is becoming a mother.

(NCT 1981).

Members of the NCT felt strongly that the Briggs Report, from the Committee on Nursing (1972), was unhelpful for mothers and for midwives. The NCT said 'It was apparent that those who had constructed the proposals had no sense of the different style of services aimed at the healthy within the community, and the services aimed at the sick in hospital (NCT 1979b).

An opportunity to influence midwives and other health professionals came in 1974 with the advent of Community Health Councils. Members were urged to apply for seats. After the Maternity Care in Action reports (Maternity Services Advisory Committee 1982/1984) members also applied to sit on local Maternity Services Liaison Committees (MSLCs). Women's experiences of trying to get MSLCs to recommend woman-centred policies have been a series of uphill struggles. User representatives have sometimes found midwives reluctant to speak up for women or for themselves (Newburn 1992). Many of the difficulties women faced were caused by the composition and functioning of the committees. The chair was often taken by an obstetrician who was unsympathetic to the involvement of user representatives and open discussion. In response to the variation between committees and the difficulties within them, the NCT issued its own *Model Terms of Reference for MSLCs* (Lewison 1994).

By the spring of 1980 the NCT Journal included the testament, 'To most NCT mothers, the midwife is the key person in their labours' (NCT 1980). There was a sense in which, for many women, a great journey had been completed; the journey from seeing the midwife as an obstacle to seeing her as a friend, advocate, comforter and source of strength. While it was acknowledged by women that the midwife was the key person in their labour – a midwife was, after all, the responsible professional present at 70% of all births – it was still a relatively novel idea that the midwife would be committed to fulfilling the woman's wishes.

MASS PROTEST

In the early 1980s birth moved once and for all from being a private experience to being a political issue. A mass public demonstration was held at the Royal Free Hospital in London in 1982 in protest at the way one obstetrician was laying down the law. Women were being told they may not deliver on the floor in a squatting position but must use the beds provided. Midwives were being told how they should and should not provide normal midwifery care. By this time, ARM was providing a support and information network. Although midwives often kept their membership a secret, those who were working for change had peers to encourage and inspire them.

In 1986 ARM published *The Vision: Proposals for the Future of the Maternity Services*. The report noted 'the strides our profession has made, particularly in the last ten years' but concluded that 'the crisis is far from over'. It went on, 'Many midwives feel frustrated with the present segmented pattern of care and find themselves feeling far from practitioners in their own right' (ARM 1986). *The Vision* set out eight basic principles which reflected and focused the views of the childbirth movement (ARM 1986). They became central to the debate in the following decade:

- that the relationship of the mother and midwife is fundamental to good midwifery care;
- that the mother is the central person in the process of care;
- informed choice in childbirth for women;
- full utilization of midwives' skills;
- continuity of care for all childbearing women;
- community-based care;
- accountability of services to those receiving them;
- care should do no harm to mother and baby.

The decade saw other important developments. *Where to be Born: The Debate and the Evidence* (Campbell and MacFarlane 1987) provided a sound critique of the policy of centralizing all births. The Association for Community-based

Maternity Care was formed. The influence of 'active birth' extended. The ideas of Janet Balaskas, Yehudi Gordon and Michel Odent caught the popular imagination. The use of yoga and water for birth preparation and pain relief became accepted as one of the range of choices available. Midwives raised funds to buy birth pools and set about teaching themselves about assisting women to give birth in water.

Caroline Flint conducted a randomized controlled trial to compare the effects for women and their babies of the 'know your midwife' scheme with those of conventional care. Iain Chalmers and Adrian Grant of the National Perinatal Epidemiology Unit supported her to use an experimental design for the research which showed convincingly that there were significant differences. There were benefits for the women who had less fragmented, more personalized care. Among other things, they needed less pain relief in labour and were more likely to feel very well prepared for looking after a baby (Flint and Poulengeris 1987). A practical guide for community midwives was written that drew on research evidence and overtly suggested midwives use research in their practice (Cronk and Flint 1989). This was becoming much easier to do following publication of a breakthrough handbook guide to systematic reviews of maternity care, which included summaries on forms of care that reduced negative outcomes, appeared promising or 'should be abandoned in the light of the evidence' (Enkin, Keirse and Chalmers 1989).

Growing numbers of midwives began to practise outside of the NHS. Working independently of the hierarchical hospital system, they were able to build a relationship with women and their families. These midwives encouraged women to make choices. They made it possible for women to choose a home birth and to receive continuity of care from one or two familiar midwives.

After becoming president of the NCT, Eileen Hutton invited members to participate in focused discussion groups where she asked them about their best and worst memories of pregnancy, labour and the early postnatal days. The importance of midwives, and the value placed on good midwifery care, came through very clearly. The women who had known their midwives before going into labour said how important this had been. Those who had felt that their midwives were really interested in helping them to have the sort of birth they wanted were full of appreciation. The feeling of having a midwife's undivided attention was also appreciated. Special mention was made of midwives who had stayed beyond the end of their shift to deliver the baby (Hutton 1987).

In 1989 the NCT became involved in lobbying the health minister on the regrading of midwives. The NCT urged the then Secretary of State, David Mellor, to implement the recommendations of the Social Services Select Committee (SSSC), taking issue with his statement that 'nurses and midwives can properly and conveniently be considered together'. They explained how mothers value midwives and wish their status to be fully recognized. Unfortunately, the Government decided not to implement the recommendations of the SSSC.

In 1990 group discussions were held in NCT branches, prompted by a midwife asking what it was that the NCT wanted from midwives: 'what members wanted midwives to be'. At almost every turn, members were asking for more *time* from midwives and asking midwives to expand their role. Continuity of care during pregnancy, birth and the postnatal period was high on the list of wants, and there was considerable demand for midwives to attend for more than the first 10 postnatal days. There was a lot of enthusiasm for the midwife as the first point of contact, alongside a call for midwives to be up-to-date in their knowledge of such things as foods to avoid during pregnancy, and alternative therapies.

Women wished that the system would allow midwives to provide total antenatal care unless there was a reason to refer, and give midwives the authority to admit women to hospital. Women were asking for midwives' support with domino deliveries and home births. There were many requests that midwives be allowed to stitch episiotomies, and some wanted midwives to be permitted to handle breech births and use forceps. They also took the trouble to say that they wanted midwives to have more power and authority, a higher public profile and higher status (Hutton 1990).

MATERNITY CARE RE-EXAMINED

In 1991 the House of Commons Health Select Committee announced an enquiry into the maternity services which would focus on the care of normal women expecting healthy babies. The NCT's evidence referred repeatedly to midwives:

> *Community midwifery clinics should be established and women should be able to consult with a midwife in the community to book a home birth, without first having to be referred by her GP.*

> *Health authorities should be encouraged to set up midwifery teams to enable women to have continuity of care and to offer women the options of a home birth, GP unit, or domino delivery, or full in-patient care in a consultant unit.*

> *Midwives should be able to refer women directly for screening during pregnancy and directly to a consultant obstetrician at any time during pregnancy or labour, should a complication occur.*

Conscious attempts should be made to limit medical interventions, ensuring that the use of procedures with known adverse side-effects is made on an individual rather than a routine basis.

In fact, the NCT, AIMS and the Maternity Alliance all gave similar evidence. What united them was that they were each representing the interests of women and their families and had the same messages to convey about what women wanted. Each organization called for greater choice, continuity of carer, individualized care, and for women to be treated with greater dignity and respect. They were united in saying that midwives should be able to provide maternity care for women as professionals in their own right. Not surprisingly AIMS was most outspoken. They said, for example, 'Women should in the main receive total care from midwives. We recognize this change will be difficult to bring about because of the financial interest involved. If GPs have to be bought off to enable women to get continuity of care, so be it' (AIMS 1991).

It was a breakthrough when the Health Committee published its report in 1992, concluding that 'it was no longer acceptable that the pattern of maternity care provision should be driven by presumptions about the applicability of a medical model of care based on unproven assertions' (Health Select Committee 1992). The NCT was able for the first time to welcome a report on the maternity services warmly and almost without reservation.

Interestingly, despite the geographical distance, developments in New Zealand have been close to those in the UK. In the foreword of the Parents Centre history, the New Zealand Minister of Women's Affairs and Associate Minister of Education, Hon Margaret Shields, wrote:

It has been particularly difficult for mothers to be given the power to choose how and where and with whom in attendance they wish to give birth. This story is particularly timely given the current amendment to the Nurses Act. . . . This amendment will allow a midwife to take responsibility for the care of a woman through her pregnancy, childbirth and the post-natal period. I cannot think of a time in a woman's life when the continuity of care and the support of another woman is more important.

(Dobbie 1990)

New Zealand women achieved the vote before British women, they also organized a childbirth group some years earlier. There are now consumers on the New Zealand College of Midwives' boards of management (Parents Centre Magazine 1993). In this country there are now user representatives on the UKCC midwifery committee and the RCM breastfeeding committee. However, the Council of the Royal College of Midwives is made up wholly of midwives.

CONCLUSION

The NCT, AIMS, Maternity Alliance and others in the childbirth movement have played a significant part in bringing about change. There is a consensus among parents' organizations and midwives that maternity services should be woman-centred and that on-going care from a familiar midwife is important for all women. There is greater awareness of parents' needs. Whatever else happens in the future, the idea that users should be consulted about maternity services now seems to be accepted.

The childbirth movement identified a problem. Birth had become over-medicalized, care was fragmented and rigid, and women's needs were hardly considered. The live delivery of the baby was considered most important; the doctor was responsible for ensuring the safety of the baby, and the midwife was delegated responsibility for carrying out the doctor's orders. The mother came at the bottom of the pecking order, to do as she was told so as not to harm her baby.

Happily, that way of thinking and delivering maternity care has been held up to critical scutiny. The values on which it is based have been turned on their head. The Expert Maternity Group report, *Changing Childbirth* (1993), now government policy, acknowledges that the woman should be the central focus of care and that her individual needs should be met. The midwife is to work 'with woman', supporting her and following her; literally following her between community and hospital, and following her decisions and her feelings during pregnancy, the birth and postnatally. The doctor is to provide back-up for the midwife when a medical opinion is needed or a woman's pregnancy or labour ceases to be normal. The baby will be cared for as much by the mother as the health professionals, and they can make a positive contribution to the baby's well-being by empowering and supporting the mother.

By making the woman the centre of care rather than the baby's safety, the baby's needs are better served. For if the woman receives individualized care so does the baby. If the woman feels valued and positive about herself, she becomes a more confident and able mother (Flint 1986). Nobody wishes to protect and nurture the baby more than the parents themselves.

ACKNOWLEDGEMENT

The authors would like to thank Beverley Beech, Caroline Flint, Sheila Kitzinger, Sandar Warshal and Angela Young for talking about their recollections and understandings. They would like to thank Patricia Donnithorne,

NCT librarian and information officer for preserving archive material and for her on-going support.

NOTE ABOUT THE AUTHORS

Eileen Hutton, President of the National Childbirth Trust (1985–1995), served on the Expert Maternity Group. Mary Newburn is Head of Policy Research at the National Childbirth Trust.

REFERENCES

Allen, V. (1990) *The Legacy of Grantly Dick-Read*, London: National Childbirth Trust.

Arms, S. (1975) *Immaculate Deception: A New Look at Women and Childbirth in America*, Boston: Houghton Mifflin.

Ashford, J.R. and Fryer, J.G. (1970) Perinatal mortality, birth-weight, and place of confinement in England and Wales 1956–65. In McLachlan, G. and Shegog, R. (eds) *In the Beginning: Studies of Maternity Services*, London: Oxford University Press.

Association for Improvements in Maternity Care (1991) *Childbirth Care – Users' Views*, Submission to the House of Commons Health Committee, AIMS.

Association of Radical Midwives (1986) *The Vision: Proposals for the Future of the Maternity Services*, ARM.

Beech, B. (1981) The work of the Association for Improvement in the Maternity Services. Paper presented to 4th Human Relations in Obstetrics Seminar, University of Glasgow, 13 Sept. 1981 (unpublished).

Benyon, C.L. (1957) The normal second stage of labour, *Journal of Obstetrics and Gynaecology British Empire* **64**: 815–20.

Borton, H., Newburn, M., Moran Ellis, J. *et al.* (1989) *Rupture of the Membranes in Labour*, London: NCT.

Boyd, C. and Sellers, L. (1982) *The British Way of Birth*, London: Pan.

Briance, P. (1982) *Childbirth with Confidence*, London: The Dick-Read School for Natural Childbirth.

Briggs, A. (1972) *Report from the Committee on Nursing, CMND 5115*, London: HMSO.

Caldeyro-Barcia, R. (1979) Physiological and psychological bases for the modern and humanised management of normal labour. In *Scientific Publication no. 858*, Montevideo, Uruguay: Centro Latino Americano de Perinatologia y Desarrollo Humano.

Campbell, R. and MacFarlane, A. (1987) *Where to be Born? The Debate and the Evidence*, Oxford: National Perinatal Epidemiology Unit.

Cranbrook Report (1959) *Report of the Maternity Services Committee*, London: HMSO.

Cronk, M. and Flint, C. (1989) *Community Midwifery: A Practical Guide*, Oxford: Heinemann.

Dawson, J., Hutton, E. and Chatfield, C. (1971) *Maternity Services in Bath*, London: NCT.

Department of Health (1993) *Changing Childbirth, Report of the Expert Maternity Group*, London: HMSO.

Dick-Read, G. (1933) *Natural Childbirth*, London: Heinemann.

Dick-Read, G. (1952) *Childbirth Without Fear*, London: Heinemann.

Dobbie, M. (1990) *The Trouble with Women: The Study of Parents' Centre New Zealand*, New Zealand: Cape Catley Ltd.

Donnison, J. (1988) *Midwives and Medicine Men*, London: Heinemann.

Durward, L. and Evans, R. (1990) Pressure groups and maternity care. In Garcia, J., Kilpatrick, R. and Richards, M. (eds) *The Politics of Maternity Care*, Oxford: Clarendon Press.

Enkin, M., Keirse, M. and Chalmers, I. (1989) *A Guide to Effective Care in Pregnancy and Childbirth*, Oxford: Oxford University Press.

Flint, C. (1986) *Sensitive Midwifery*, London: Heinemann.

Flint, C. and Poulengeris, P. (1987) *Know your Midwife Report*, Pub. 49, Peckerman's Wood, London SE26 6RZ.

Gaskin, I.M. and the Farm Midwives (1975) *Spiritual Midwifery*, Summertown, USA: Tenn Book Publishing Company.

Goodman, M. (1994) *Mothers' Pride and Others' Prejudice*, London: Maternity Alliance.

Halle, M. (1994) GP takes the plunge and tries an underwater birth, *GP*, 20 May, 1994.

Green, J., Coupland, V. and Kitzinger, J. (1988) *Great Expectations: A Prospective Study of Women's Expectations and Experiences of Childbirth*, Cambridge: Childcare and Development Group, University of Cambridge.

Greenshields, W. (1988) *Postnatal Infection*, London: NCT.

Greenshields, W. and Hulme, H. (1993) *The Perineum in Childbirth*, London: National Childbirth Trust.

Haire, D. (1972) *The Cultural Warping of Childbirth*, International Childbirth Education Association, USA.

Haire, D. (1984) Fetal effects of ultrasound: a growing controversy, *Nurse-Midwifery* **29(4):** 241–6.

Health Select Committee (1992) *Second Report on the Maternity Services*, London: HMSO.

Hould, S. (1988) Midwives in Denmark. In Kitzinger, K. (ed.) *The Midwife Challenge*, London: Pandora.

Hutton, E. (1987) 'Having a baby now', *New Generation*, Vol. 6, No. 2, June, pp. 6–7.

Hutton, E. (1990) 'What do you want from midwives', *New Generation*, Vol. 9, No. 4, December, pp. 5–6.

Inch, S. (1982) *Birthrights: A Parents' Guide to Modern Childbirth*, London: Hutchinson.

International Childbirth Education Association (1966) *Convention Report*, ICEA, USA.

Katz Rothman, B. (1982) *In Labour: Women and Power in the Birth Place*, London: Junction Books.

Kirkham, M. (1989) Midwives and information giving during labour. In Robinson, S. and Thomson, A.M. (eds) *Midwives, Research and Childbirth Vol. 1*, London: Chapman & Hall.

Kitzinger, J. (1990) Strategies of the early childbirth movement: a case study of the National Childbirth Trust. In Garcia, J. Kilpatrick, R. and Richards, M. (eds) *The Politics of Maternity Care*, Oxford: Clarendon Press.

Kitzinger, S. (1962) *The Experience of Childbirth*, London: Gollancz.

Kitzinger, S. (1975) *Some Women's Experiences of Induced Labour*, London: NCT.

Kitzinger, S. (1978) *Women as Mothers*, London: Collins.

Kitzinger, S. (1979a) *Birth at Home, 1979*, Oxford: Oxford University Press.

Kitzinger, S. (1979b) *The Experience of Breastfeeding*, Harmondsworth: Pelican.

Kitzinger, S. (1979c) *The Good Birth Guide*, London: Fontana.

Kitzinger, S. (1983a) *The New Good Birth Guide*, Harmondsworth: Penguin.

Kitzinger, S. (1983b) *Woman's Experience of Sex*, London: Dorling Kindersley.

Kitzinger, S. (1987) *Some Women's Experience of Epidural*, London: NCT.

Kitzinger, S. (1988) *The Midwife Challenge*, London: Pandora.

Kitzinger, S. and Davis, J. (1978) *The Place of Birth*, Oxford: Oxford University Press.

Kitzinger, S. and Walters, R. (1981) *Some Women's Experience of Episiotomy*, London: NCT.

Leap, N. and Hunter, B. (1993) *The Midwife's Tale*, London: Scarlett Press.

Lewis, J. (1990) Mothers and maternity policies in the twentieth century. In Garcia, J., Kilpatrick, R. and Richards, M. (eds) *The Politics of Maternity Care*, Oxford: Clarendon Press.

Lewison, H. (1994) *Model Terms of Reference for MSLCs*, London: GLACHC and NCT.

Maternity Alliance (1989) *Changing Childbirth: Interventions in Labour in England and Wales*, London: Maternity Alliance.

Maternity Services Advisory Committee (1982/4) *Maternity Care in Action Part I Antenatal Care (1982), and Part II Care During Childbirth (Intrapartum) Care (1984)*, London: HMSO.

Mickelthwait, P., Beard, R. and Shaw, K. (1978) Expectations of a pregnant woman in relation to her treatment, *British Medical Journal* 2: 118–19.

Midwives Chronicle (1992) *The Maternity Services Report*, October, pp. 314–15.

Mitford, J. (1993) *The American Way of Birth*, London: Gollancz.

National Childbirth Trust (1960) *Labour*, London: NCT.

National Childbirth Trust (1962) *Exercises and Posture During Pregnancy*, London: NCT.

National Childbirth Trust (1964a) *Breathing During Labour*, London: NCT.

National Childbirth Trust (1964b) *Caring for the New Baby*, London: NCT.

National Childbirth Trust (1966) *The Helpers Handbook*, London: NCT.

National Childbirth Trust (1968a) *Why Breastfeed?* London: NCT.

National Childbirth Trust (1968b) *Annual Report*, London: NCT.

National Childbirth Trust (1974a) *Newsletter 25*, Autumn, p. 16, London: NCT.

National Childbirth Trust (1974b) *Annual Report*, London: NCT.

National Childbirth Trust (1978) *Journal*, Spring, pp. 20–1, London: NCT.

National Childbirth Trust (1979a) *Teachers' Broadsheet*, Vol. 2, London: NCT.

National Childbirth Trust (1979b) *Journal*, Spring 1979, p. 17, London: NCT.

National Childbirth Trust (1980a) *Response to the Parliamentary Social Services Committee on Perinatal and Neonatal Mortality*, unpublished.

National Childbirth Trust (1980b) *Journal*, Spring, London: NCT.

National Childbirth Trust (1981) *Report of the NCT Working Party on Antenatal Care*, unpublished.

National Childbirth Trust (1991) *Maternity Services Survey*, unpublished.

National Childbirth Trust (1992) *Maternity Services Survey*, London: NCT.

Newburn, M. (1992) Participation in policy-making: the maternity service users. In Chamberlain, G. and Zander, L. (eds) *Pregnancy Care in the 1990s*, Carnforth: Parthenon.

Newburn, M. (1993) 'Choice, Continuity and Care', *New Generation*, June.

NHS Management Executive (1992) *Local Voices*, NHSME.

Nursing Times, Correspondence, 10 November 1977.

Nursing Times, Correspondence, 1 December 1977.

Nursing Times, Correspondence, 12 January 1978.

Oakley, A. (1984) *The Captured Womb*, Oxford: Blackwell.

Oakley, A. and Houd, S. (1990) *Helpers in Childbirth: Midwifery Today*, London: Hemisphere Publishing.

Page, L. (1988) The midwife's role in modern health care. In Kitzinger, S. (ed.) *The Midwife Challenge*, London: Pandora.

Parents Centre Magazine, Vol. 138, September/October 1993.

Peel Report (1970) *Domiciliary Midwifery and Maternity Bed Needs*, Report of the Sub-Committee, Central Health Services Council Standing Maternity and Midwifery Advisory Committee, London: HMSO.

Roberts, E. (1984) *A Woman's Place: An Oral History of Working Class Women 1890–1940*, London: Blackwell.

Romney, M. (1980) Predelivery shaving: an unjustified assault? *Journal of Obstetrics and Gynaecology* **1**: 33–5.

Romney, M. and Gordon, H. (1981) Is your enema really necessary? *British Medical Journal*, **282:** 1269–71.

Short Report (1980) *Perinatal and Neonatal Mortality*, Second Report from the Parliamentry Social Services Committee 1979–80, London: HMSO.

Smith, A. (1970) Progress in the 1960s and Problems for the 1970s. In McLachlan, G. and Shegog, R. (eds) *In the Beginning: Studies of Maternity Services*, London: Oxford University Press.

Sousa, M. (1976) *Childbirth at Home*, Englewood Cliffs, USA: Prentice Hall.

Stewart, D. and Stewart, L. (eds) (1976) *Safe Alternatives in Childbirth*, NAPSAC, USA.

Tew, M. (1977) 'Where to be Born?', *New Society*, Vol. 39.

Wagner, M. (1994) *Pursuing the Birth Machine*, London: ACE Graphics.

Watson, V. (1994) 'Maternal Position in the Second Stage of Labour', *Modern Midwife*, July.

World Health Organization (1985) *Having a Baby in Europe*, Geneva: WHO.

Index

Note: as references to midwifery and maternity services are ubiquitous, these terms have largely been omitted as qualifiers.